# A
# MOTOR RELEARNING PROGRAMME
# FOR STROKE

# A
# Motor Relearning Programme
# for Stroke

## Janet H. Carr

*Fellow of the Australian College of Physiotherapists;*
*Lecturer, School of Physiotherapy, Cumberland*
*College of Health Sciences, Sydney, Australia.*

## Roberta B. Shepherd

*Fellow of the Australian College of Physiotherapists;*
*Senior Lecturer, School of Physiotherapy, Cumberland*
*College of Health Sciences, Sydney, Australia.*

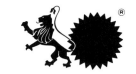

AN ASPEN PUBLICATION
Aspen Systems Corporation
Rockville, Maryland
London
1983

Printed in Great Britain

# Contents

# *Preface*

This book comprises a motor relearning programme (MRP) for stroke. In addition, some guidelines are given for establishing an environment which is conducive to learning and in which the person, following stroke, can make his best possible recovery of function. Appendices outline the factors which seem particularly essential for motor training, and indicate the theoretical mechanisms by which recovery may take place.

The MRP emphasises specific training of motor control in everyday activities, commenced as soon as the person's medical condition is stable. It represents a shift away from facilitation of movement and exercise therapy and involves specific training of muscle activity and functional movement of the affected limbs and the prevention of compensatory activity by either the affected or the intact side. The Programme's success depends upon the therapist training the patient to activate muscles in exactly the way they perform in normal everyday functions, monitoring his performance so the patient knows what he should and should not practise, preventing the habituation of incorrect motor responses. The techniques used require the patient to concentrate and to use his cognitive abilities, and side effects of the Programme have been improved concentration and cognitive function.

The development of this Programme represents the culmination of extensive literature research together with several years of clinical and teaching experience. We are aware of the need to research thoroughly the effectiveness of any new developments in physiotherapy, particularly since the therapeutic measures at present employed in stroke re-habilitation are carried out despite there having been little or no investigation of their effectiveness. In determining how to do this research, we had two objectives in mind. The first was to write out our treatment ideas in detail as a specific Programme so we would know exactly what we were researching. A problem in researching existing methods of treatment is their lack of detailed documentation. The second was to develop an assessment tool, since we considered that no existing instrument would adequately measure the most essential motor functions. We therefore set about the two tasks. This book is the result of the first. A motor assessment scale* for stroke which has been tested and found to have both inter-rater reliability and test-retest reliability is the result of the second.

Our clinical experience and that of several colleagues using this

*Carr J. H., Lynne, D., Nordholm L., Shepherd R. B. (1982). A Motor Assessment Scale for Stroke. *Proceedings of the IXth WCPT Congress, Stockholm.*

Programme have been so encouraging that we feel justified in publishing the Programme before it has been researched. This research will commence with a series of single-person case studies. The MRP in its present state represents a beginning of what we consider will constitute a new direction in physiotherapy for the person with brain damage. It is our intention to continue the Programme's development as increasing knowledge and the results of research enable us to make changes and additions. We hope others will also be interested in developing these ideas further.

The MRP appears prescriptive in terms of the treatment or training given. However, the choice of movement components on which to concentrate, the monitoring of the patient's performance and the increasing of complexity will depend on the individual therapist analysing problems accurately and thoroughly and making the correct decisions. The individuality of patients is often used as a reason for not developing prescriptive programmes, for not researching treatment and to support the existence of many different treatment 'approaches'. However, although patients are indeed individuals, the basic motor needs of all humans are the same and our methods of learning motor skills have many common aspects. The existence of many different 'approaches' in stroke rehabilitation may indicate that none is truly effective and the idea that a variety of different approaches to treatment is advantageous or necessary is probably misleading.

We have not set out to write a complete book on stroke. The MRP represents the physiotherapist's contribution to the rehabilitation process in terms of motor training and, to be fully effective, the Programme will need to be combined with other planned programmes for stimulating mental, communication, visual and other functions. There should be easy access to medical care, psychiatric care and community resources. The patient must be in an environment in which motivation, positive attitudes, reinforcement from relatives and friends and consistency of practice are organised, not left to chance or to the goodwill of staff.

Extensive referencing has been included throughout the text in order that interested therapists and others may read the material which has helped us develop our theories and in order to encourage research into the many questions this Programme raises. Throughout the Programme, as in the rest of this book, the masculine pronoun refers to the patient and the feminine to the therapist, except in the captions to the photographs, when the pronoun will relate directly to the person photographed.

# Acknowledgements

The authors wish particularly to thank David Robinson who took the photographs and Sue Ferris, assisted by Therese Adams, who typed the manuscript.

For their valuable comments and suggestions we wish to thank, in Australia, Louise Ada, Roger Adams, Ron Balnave, Colleen Canning, Dave Sanderson and Pippa Warrell; and in North America, John Basmajian, Leonard Diller, Richard Herman, Ron Marteniuk, Eric Roy, Shirley Sahrmann, Shirley Stockmeyer, Edward Taub, Paul Wang, and those masters, doctoral and post-doctoral students at Columbia University, New York and the University of Waterloo who gave their time and thought to discussing our ideas with us. Our grateful thanks go also to the people whose photographs appear throughout the text.

Figures 3.2 and 3.3 are from *Physiotherapy in Disorders of the Brain* (Janet H. Carr and Roberta B. Shepherd, 1980) published by William Heinemann Medical Books Ltd. Figure 3.4 is reproduced with permission from the *Australian Journal of Physiotherapy*.

In conclusion, we would also like to express our thanks to the Principal of Cumberland College of Health Sciences, Dr Jeffrey Miller, and the College Council who granted us three months leave, and to Doreen Moore, the Head of the School of Physiotherapy, for her support and encouragement.

# PART I

# 1

# *Background to the development of the MRP*

Although stroke rehabilitation has to some extent progressed over the years, there is still a lack of enthusiasm in pursuing the goal of ensuring that each patient recovers his best possible function. The **quality** of rehabilitation must be questioned since much of it is based on outdated ideas of exercise therapy, negative expectations, and on the supposed need to **wait** for recovery to occur. The major objective in the early stages is still expressed as the prevention of contractures when it should instead be the active stimulation of muscle activity and the training of motor control in activities relevant to daily life.

For these reasons the contribution of physiotherapy as expressed in the literature is still unclear. Some studies,[1,2] for example, have shown that the results following simple functional care are similar to the results following formal rehabilitation. One study[3] found that pain and stiffness in the shoulder developed more commonly in patients who received physiotherapy than in those who did not. Unfortunately, results from studies such as these detract from the potential contribution of physiotherapy following stroke. Physiotherapy itself falls into disrepute, when it is the choice of methods which has been at fault.

Therapists still follow therapeutic concepts developed three decades ago, although these have never been developed and written down in a manner which enables them to be tested for effectiveness. Effort is expended in comparing these concepts and in developing an eclectic approach which can embrace all of them,[4] with the result that physiotherapy gives the appearance of looking backwards rather than forward, and of being more interested in techniques of treatment than in analysing the motor problems. This effort would be better spent in developing new concepts more in keeping with modern knowledge. Theoretical considerations still seem to depend solely on neurophysiological data despite the advances in knowledge made by biomechanists and behavioural scientists. And, by and large, although many patients return home following stroke, the accepted norms in terms of motor function are walking deficiencies which require an aid of some sort and a non-functional upper extremity. In other words, the end result of a patient's lengthy rehabilitation process is frequently disabilities which may have been to some extent augmented by the very procedures intended to overcome

3

these disabilities. The authors' clinical experience is that the end result of rehabilitation can be very different, but that this depends on physiotherapists recognising the real potential of physiotherapy, discarding ineffective methods, understanding the need to develop new methods of treatment, researching their effectiveness and taking more responsibility for improving the general framework of stroke care.

Motor control is essential to almost every aspect of life, and the unique contribution of physiotherapy to the rehabilitation of stroke lies potentially in the retraining of motor control based on an understanding of normal movement and an analysis of the motor dysfunction.

For a number of years the authors have been working to develop what they consider should be the direction of modern stroke rehabilitation, a major shift in emphasis away from exercise therapy to the relearning of motor control. This new direction has, to some extent, its origins in the work of K. and B. Bobath who pointed out the need for treatment to be directly related to functional activities, the importance of gaining control over antigravity responses and the need to control excessive muscle activity.

However, the material from which this motor relearning programme has most recently been derived comes not from medical or physiotherapy literature but from studies of human movement and motor skill acquisition and theories of learning and motivation. Emphasis in the Programme is on practice of specific activities, the training of cognitive control over muscles and over the movement components of these activities, together with conscious elimination of all muscle activity which is unnecessary. Rehabilitation therefore involves the relearning of real-life activities, those which have meaning for the patient, not the practice of exercises.

At present, physiotherapy for stroke varies not only from hospital to hospital but also from therapist to therapist within the same hospital and this is no doubt one of the reasons why it is unusual to see the details of treatment written down and why the few studies done to evaluate effectiveness and outcome omit these details. Yet, if effectiveness is ever to be evaluated and if more appropriate methods of treatment are ever to enter into general use, treatment programmes must be described in detail. Of course, there are subtleties in physical treatment which are difficult to describe and some of these have to do with the therapist herself, her personality, her attitudes and her abilities. Physiotherapists have for too long used the fact that each patient needs individual treatment to excuse the lack of research into the effectiveness of treatment. Although treatment must take into account the needs of the individual patient, all stroke patients who have motor problems lack the essential movement components of activities such as standing up and walking, and therefore have the same basic motor needs. Experience with a large number of people following stroke has led the authors to the conclusion that it would be possible to design and write out a programme around a framework of these basic motor needs from which all patients would benefit, and which could be tested for effectiveness.

Compared with the prevailing rehabilitation attitudes, the MRP appears prescriptive. However, looked at closely it will be seen to depend upon the therapist's analysis of her patient's problems. Once each problem has been analysed and the therapist has made the necessary decisions, the Programme prescribes the methodology, that is, the training regime.

The Programme assumes the brain's capacity for **reorganisation and adaptation** and is aimed at either stimulating this or making the best possible use of it, or both. Appendix 1 gives details of current theories of the mechanisms by which adaptation may take place.

The Programme is based on three factors known to be essential for the learning of motor skill and therefore assumed to be essential for the relearning of motor control following stroke: the **elimination of unnecessary muscle activity, feedback** and **practice**. Appendices 2, 3 and 4 give some details relating to these three factors.

A motor skill has been defined as 'any human activity that has become better organised and more effective as a result of practice'.[5] Everyday activities, even such apparently simple ones as standing up from sitting, therefore constitute motor skills. These activities are made up of movement components which, when linked together correctly, allow smooth, controlled movement. Some components are more essential to the activity than others and are called biomechanical necessities[6] or determinants[7] as they are the key elements upon which the activity depends. Hence, it is theorised that if the patient learns to perform these components and to perform them in a controlled manner and in the correct sequence, he will be able to perform the entire activity. The Programme is organised in such a way as to enable the therapist to train the patient to perform the key components which are missing and to follow this with practice of the entire activity.

Relearning the everyday activities contained in this Programme appears to involve the patient remembering the movements in which he was skilled before his stroke, helped by therapy which triggers off previously learned motor programmes (engrams), and which trains the muscular activity necessary for these movements. In training muscular activity, the therapist must take into account the complexity of muscle function, something which traditional exercise therapy and many so-called neurophysiological techniques do not do. Muscles can change function (for example, from rotation to flexion) depending on the initial position of the body part and the action which is being carried out,[8] that is, relative activity of particular muscles differs in different actions.[9]

The mechanical response of a muscle to a neural signal appears to depend on the mechanical condition of the muscle at the moment the signal arrives. A motor activity is therefore affected by such peripheral factors as muscle length, velocity, temperature, joint angle, length of limb segments and external forces.[10] The warm-up phenomenon suggests that muscles may contract more efficiently after they have contracted a few times thereby producing heat. It is possible that the nervous system may be able to take advantage of certain muscle properties in order to use more easily generated neural signals to accomplish the desired result.[10] The aim in motor training is not *muscle strength* but *muscle control*. That is, the therapist aims not at the activation of a maximum number of motor units but at helping the patient control the activity of the appropriate number of motor units for the particular function being retrained.

Necessary for all motor activity is the body's ability to **adjust to gravity**, so throughout practice of all activities, the therapist monitors the alignment of the body and the patient is trained to preserve a balanced alignment as he moves about. Missing components of alignment are practised specifically when necessary. Appendix 5 gives some details related to normal balance.

Throughout the Programme, emphasis is on the patient using cognitive functions in the initial stages of learning, progressing to practice at a more automatic level in order to ensure that skill has been acquired. It is possible that the emphasis placed on cognitive function and on learning[11] is itself an important stimulation to brain recovery. The authors' experience with people in the very early stages following stroke is that the stimulus to thinking provided by the Programme results in a marked and swift increase in alertness and motivation. Blood-flow studies[12,13] show that there is an increase in blood flow of approximately 20% when a subject is thinking.

If the patient is to learn, the rehabilitation environment must encourage the learning process. The therapist must take the responsibility for creating the right environment for recovery and for learning and should liaise with the rest of the rehabilitation team in ensuring a positive milieu. These points are further elaborated in Chapter 2 of this section.

In order to use the Programme effectively, the therapist must develop her problem-solving skills. Problem-solving can be divided into five stages: recognition, analysis, decision-making, action-taking, and re-evaluation. Of these, the analysis and decision-making stages are probably the most crucial, and it is in these that most errors in therapeutic problem-solving occur. The MRP gives some guidance in problem analysis, but effective analysis must depend upon the individual therapist's knowledge of movement. The therapist with a limited understanding of muscle action and movement will be unable to make a correct analysis of problems and this will result in inappropriate decisions about treatment which may not only be ineffective but may actually worsen the problems or initiate a new problem.

Here are two examples of inadequate analysis leading to incorrect decision-making and therefore to inappropriate action-taking.

1. Difficulty stepping forward with the affected leg may be incorrectly analysed as being due to 'foot drop'. The patient may, as a result, be trained to hitch his hip during swing phase in order to clear his foot from the ground. However, difficulty clearing the foot from the ground during swing phase is usually due to a lack of knee flexion at toe-off and not to lack of dorsiflexion. Therapy should therefore be directed at stimulating knee flexor activity at the particular point (the initiation of swing phase) when it should normally occur (see p. 133).

2. Analysis of a person who has movement problems may reveal that he has a lack of awareness of proprioceptive and tactile sensations on the affected side. If the therapist decides that movement difficulties are due principally to sensory dysfunction, she may commence the patient on a

programme of sensory stimulation. However, the sensory unawareness may be due principally to lack of use of the affected limbs, and a more appropriate decision would be, in this case, to institute a motor programme in which the patient has the chance to regain sensory awareness through practice of movements which emphasise the affected side of the body.

However, a person who is regaining effective hand function may not be progressing in activities which require fine handling because of a degree of insensitivity at his fingertips. In this case, sensory acuity can be developed by, for example, practice of two-point discrimination, games involving recognition of texture and objects, as well as by practice in manipulating objects which require a fine degree of skill. In this case, the decision to include sensory stimulation (specific stimulation, not generalised) would be correct.

The effectiveness of the MRP depends to a large extent on the ability of the individual therapist:

- to recognise and analyse the problem

- to select the most essential missing movement components

- to explain clearly to the patient by speech and demonstration

- to monitor the patient's performance and give verbal feedback

- to re-evaluate throughout each session the effectiveness of her own and the patient's performance

- to progress the patient's level of performance as soon as he has grasped the idea of what he is practising

- to ensure a positive milieu with consistency of practice throughout the patient's day

- to provide an enriched environment in which the patient will be motivated towards recovery of both mental and physical abilities.

## REFERENCES

1. Feldman D. J., Unterecker J., Lloyd K., Rusk H. A. and Toole A. (1962). A comparison of functionally orientated medical care and formal rehabilitation in the management of patients with hemiplegia due to cerebrovascular disease. *J. chron. Dis*; **15**:297–310.
2. Stern P. H., McDowell F., Miller J. M. and Robinson M. (1971). Factors influencing stroke rehabilitation. *Stroke*; **2**:213.
3. Brocklehurst J. C., Andrews K., Richards B. and Laycock P. J. (1978). How much physical therapy following stroke? *Brit. med. J*; 20 May:1307–1310.
4. Cocke M., Sawner K. A. and Scheer K. (1981). An integrated treatment approach to adult hemiplegia: Brunnstrom approach, neurodevelopmental treatment, proprioceptive neuromuscular facilitation technique. Unpublished paper delivered at *Annual Congress of APTA, Washington*.
5. Annett J. (1971). Acquisition of skill. *Brit. med. Bull*; **27**:266–71.

6. Broer M. R. and Zernicke R. F. (1979). *Efficiency of Human Movement*, 4th edn. Philadelphia: Saunders.

7. Saunders J. B., Inman V. T. and Eberhart H. D. (1953). The major determinants in normal and pathological gait. *J. Bone Jt Surg;* **35A, 3**:543–58.

8. Evans W. F. (1976). *Anatomy and Physiology*, 2nd edn. New Jersey: Prentice-Hall.

9. Alexander R. McN. (1975). Evolution of integrated design. *Amer. Zool;* **15**:419–25.

10. Partridge L. D. (1979). Muscle properties: a problem for the motor controller physiologist. In *Posture and Movement* (Talbott R. E. and Humphrey D. R. eds.) pp. 189–229. New York: Raven Press.

11. Rosenzweig M. R. (1980). Responsiveness of brain size to individual experience: behavioral and evolutionary implications. In *Development and Evolution of Brain Size: Behavioral Implications* (Hahn M., Jensen C. and Dudek B. eds.) New York: Academic Press.

12. Ingvor D. H. and Philipson L. (1977). Distribution of cerebral blood flow in the dominant hemisphere during motor ideation and motor performance. *Ann. Neurol;* **2**:230–37.

13. Yonekura M. (1981). Evaluation of cerebral blood flow in patients with transient attacks and minor strokes. *J. surg. Neurol;* **15**:58–65.

# 2

## *Creating the right environment for recovery and for learning*

The purpose of rehabilitation should be to provide an environment for the patient in which he can learn how to regain motor control, reasoning ability and social skills. The MRP will have its maximum effectiveness if it is part of a rehabilitation environment in which there can be consistency of practice and the opportunity for personal development. In this chapter the authors suggest the conditions which are necessary for learning to take place, which will best stimulate the brain to adapt and re-organise and which will ensure generalisation or transfer of learning from the rehabilitation setting into everyday life. Insufficient consideration has been given in the past to the need to provide an environment for learning. It is probable that some of the failure of modern rehabilitation for stroke is due to the impoverished, non-challenging environment in which many patients find themselves.

### ADMISSION AND REFERRAL

'Stroke is a medical emergency which requires accurate diagnosis and optimum care and this can be best given in hospital.'[1]

Although there appears to be a great deal of evidence which supports admission to hospital and rehabilitation following stroke,[2-7] there are still many patients who are not admitted, whose relatives are expected to care for them at home. The stroke patient should have access to specialised diagnostic skill as well as to medical skill to reduce the incidence of complications, and this should apply as much to the elderly person as to a younger person. Without appropriate medical care an elderly person, who may otherwise have made a good recovery, may die as a result of neglect of a treatable medical problem, such as respiratory infection.

There are probably several reasons why many stroke patients are not referred for rehabilitation. Feigenson[8] includes the following in his list: many **physicians are reluctant** to treat vigorously elderly patients who have multiple medical problems; **physicians are frequently sceptical** about the effectiveness of rehabilitation on the problems following stroke; there is a **lack of facilities** adequately equipped for such rehabilitation.

The reasons for negative attitudes towards stroke amongst health professionals would be interesting to investigate. They may, for example, reflect pessimistic views about patient recovery following stroke expressed many years previously during undergraduate training.

The **cost of stroke rehabilitation**, which is high, may be another reason for non-referral, despite the fact that the cost of maintenance in the dependent state which may otherwise result is much higher.[9-11]

The effect of non-admission upon the patient and his family can be profound. Relatives can be so affected by the shock and struggle of the first few days that they may thereafter be unable and unwilling to cope with the situation. The shock associated with stroke is extreme, both for the patient and his relatives. Relatives often have great difficulty coping both emotionally and physically with the problems which arise. It may be impossible for inexperienced people to cope with their own stress as well as with the patient's stress reactions. It may also be impossible for a relative to care physically for the patient, that is, to wash and toilet him, to sit him up and to get him out of bed. The patient's feelings of helplessness and dependence are aggravated by this situation, whereas admission to an appropriate hospital unit is reassuring in its obvious provision of skilled care.

## STROKE UNITS

Several authors[12-17] support the idea that patients following stroke should be admitted to a stroke unit (a disability-oriented unit). Although there is in general an awareness that certain patients, for example the spinal cord injured, require specially trained nurses, medical practitioners and therapists, this awareness has not as yet extended to the stroke patient, who is still admitted to a general ward in the care of staff who have little understanding of his needs and, often, a pessimistic attitude towards his potential for recovery. This factor may be another reason for the poor result of rehabilitation.

It is unfortunate that many health professionals fail to appreciate the special needs of the stroke patient and because of a lack of understanding of brain function are unable to analyse his problems. Instead they may take the most obvious and superficial view of his behaviour. For example, if the patient does not do as he is asked he may be labelled 'difficult', 'unco-operative' or 'disoriented'. Analysis of his behaviour, however, may reveal that he has a unilateral spatial neglect, that competing auditory inputs with which he cannot cope result in an extinction of the input on one side, that he is profoundly depressed, and so on. A negative attitude towards the potential of people following stroke prevails in the medical, therapy and nursing professions. This is illustrated by the tendency to give custodial care rather than stimulation based on the individual's need, and physical treatment based on ideas developed 30 years ago rather than treatment which takes into account recent advances in the physiological and behavioural sciences.

Stroke units have the advantage of concentrating staff skills and interests in a collaboration which ensures a better quality of patient care.[18]

In a study[19] carried out in an attempt to determine whether or not stroke units can affect outcome, two groups of patients on similar therapeutic programmes were compared. The data showed that the stroke unit group, despite the fact that they had more medical problems and more severe neurological and functional deficits, were more likely to go home after treatment and walked better at the time they were discharged.

## THE QUALITY OF REHABILITATION

Whether or not rehabilitation is carried out within a regional stroke unit or a rehabilitation unit within an acute care hospital, it is the quality of rehabilitation which is important. There are several factors which affect the quality and therefore the outcome of rehabilitation. These include the following.

1. **An early start.** Rehabilitation should commence early,[11,18,20,21] as soon as the patient is medically stable, which is usually within 24 to 36 hours, and this should involve the patient getting out of bed and standing. There is evidence that good mental health is promoted by encouragement towards normal activities and interests,[22] and this encouragement should begin early in order to prevent a secondary mental deterioration. There are many physiological reasons also for an early start to rehabilitation, and these have to do with the brain's capacity for recovery (see Appendix 1). Stroke care begun late is inefficient and this inefficiency also adds to the cost of rehabilitation.[9]

2. **A rehabilitation plan.** This should consist of a general programme planned for all patients following stroke (involving, for example, encouragement of socialisation and communication), plus specific programmes planned to overcome particular problems.

The general programme is concerned with the way the patient spends his day, his milieu or surroundings. This ensures the provision of an appropriate environment in which the patient can be rehabilitated to his fullest potential. As soon as his vital signs are stable he should get up and dressed. Within the first week his day is planned to approximate to a normal routine: up in the morning; meals at a table with others; short nap in the afternoon; activities throughout the day, that is, times set aside for specific rehabilitation programmes and recreational activities; and to bed again, not in the late afternoon which is often the case, but at 9.00 or 10.00 p.m., following some after-dinner recreational activity.

Specific programmes are planned for each person's needs, and may include a motor programme with the physiotherapist, and a self-care programme (including dressing) with the occupational therapist. The speech pathologist will plan the means by which communication can be established and stimulated in a dysphasic patient. The neuropsychologist will plan programmes for overcoming specific visual problems, problems of neglect or of mental functioning. General relaxation training may need to be organised for the anxious or tense person.

The patient should be doing something physically and mentally for most of the day and must not spend long periods doing nothing, in isolated or depressing surroundings. Restriction of activity is known to cause impaired intellectual functioning.[23,24] The patient's day is planned, therefore, to avoid both disorientation in time and place, and helplessness.[25] Activities are planned carefully so they are enjoyable and not passive or meaningless. They should stimulate cognitive functioning and require from the patient responses to challenges similar to those he would normally receive in daily life. For example, he should gradually be encouraged to take responsibility for keeping his various appointments. He should also be encouraged to take an active part in the planning of his daily programme, stating his preferences and actually helping with the organisation.

Staff should not see themselves as merely providing custodial care but should organise actively the patient's return to normal life. Relatives, friends or volunteer helpers[26] should be involved as they will very often be more successful than health personnel at thinking of activities which simulate normal life and therefore which give the patient something familiar with which to grapple.

3. **Consistency of goals.** Time spent in individual therapy sessions without reinforcement throughout the rest of the day should be considered as time wasted. Similarly, different and contradictory methods of rehabilitation will not only be confusing but will actually *prevent* the patient from learning.

Consistency is a difficult point to establish. Learning requires the opportunity for correct practice. When the therapist is teaching the patient how to stand up (see p. 98), he will only learn this activity if he is able to practise it throughout the day. He will have a tendency to stand up with his weight on his intact leg, because of difficulty controlling his affected leg, and if the nursing staff, for example, reinforce this, it will become an habitual or learned response, and will prevent the patient regaining motor control. If, however, the nursing staff reinforce the method being taught by the therapist, *this* will become the learned response and will enable the patient to take advantage of improved motor control.

The therapist herself has to take care not to be inconsistent. She must not allow the patient to move about by pivoting on his intact leg, but should make sure he practises what he has been learning. In this way he is 'drilled' to perform correctly. Unfortunately, in the attempt to help the patient become independent, staff may encourage ways of achieving particular objectives which will actually prevent him from relearning effective function and therefore from becoming really independent. For example, a person who is encouraged to propel a wheelchair with his intact limbs may gain 'independence' of a sort. However, this activity, by encouraging the use of excessive muscular activity (associated movements), and by encouraging non-use, will probably prevent the regaining of function in the affected limbs and eventual attainment of real independence.

4. **Motivation.** One of the objectives for the physiotherapist is to plan an enriched physical and emotional environment which will motivate the patient towards recovery. There is evidence that an enriched environment may play a significant part in recovery from brain damage.[24,27,28]

Motivation needs to be organised. It may be lacking if the patient is fearful, anxious, apathetic or depressed. To benefit from his rehabilitation programme the patient must be able to learn and it is well know that little learning takes place in the absence of motivation. Many stroke patients need closer personal contact with staff than is usual in the hospital or rehabilitation setting in order to participate fully in their treatment programmes.

The patient needs to be involved in the planning of his treatment and in the discussion of treatment goals. The weekly timetable should be discussed and written up in consultation with the patient and his relatives. The plan should appear to be achievable to the patient, with goals that are understandable and immediately relevant to his needs. On the whole, training will not be effective unless there is a feeling of need for or desire to learn the particular skill involved. All patients following stroke have two major objectives—to walk and to use both hands. Part of the effectiveness of the MRP may be attributable to the motivating effect of its emphasis on directly training the patient for these functions, in contrast to exercises and activities which have no apparent relevance.

To make the best possible recovery, the patient will need to have people around him from whom he can draw courage. Staff who are stuffy, silent, aloof or too protective may actually prevent the patient from tapping his personal resources.[29] He needs reassurance, encouragement and proof of his capacity to gradually overcome the barriers with which he is surrounded.[22] Belmont and his co-workers[30] comment that brain-damaged patients probably require unique motivating conditions for performance and point out that this has received too little consideration.

Motivation can also be provided by success, reward, by positive reinforcement such as praise or an attitude of pleasure, and by receiving immediate feedback of performance.

**Success** in treatment sessions counteracts the tendency towards depression following stroke[31] as well as leading to a more rapid development of skill. The effective therapist ensures that the patient always completes an activity successfully, by monitoring his performance and giving him guidance when necessary, and by ensuring that he does not persistently attempt something he cannot do. The authors' clinical observations indicate that success is particularly important in the early stages of relearning a motor activity as it increases the patient's level of aspiration. The therapist should scale, chart or videotape the patient's performance so as to show him his improvement, as he may like to see proof of his progress.

**Positive reinforcement** is given through praise, affection and acceptance. The therapist should think carefully about the impact of praising a performance so that the patient can relate words of praise, such as 'good', to success. 'Good' is offered as a **reward** and not said automatically and without relevance. If he is not successful, the therapist can use other words or gestures in order to encourage him and to acknowledge his efforts. Praise as a direct reward is only effective if it is offered for accomplishment of some specific desired behaviour. It loses its impact if given lightly with no relationship to success.

**Social isolation** can affect the outcome of rehabilitation by affecting motivation. Hyman,[32] following an examination of the literature for some possible links between social isolation and poor performance in rehabilitation, lists ten hypotheses. These include: dissatisfaction with the pre-morbid life situation; the seeking of substitute social satisfaction in the treatment centre; lack of social support; absence of an advocate; recent bereavement; a low level of pre-morbid functioning.

If a patient appears unmotivated, the cause of this should be investigated. A patient's behaviour is a consequence of the limitations imposed on him by the damage to his brain, which results in disturbances of body responses, perceptual and thinking processes, a slowness in registering and retaining recent information, an inability to give proper language expression to what he does perceive, combined with emotional turmoil.[18] He may have difficulty grasping all aspects of a task or sorting out the essentials of a problem. The dysphasic person may have difficulty shifting mentally from one idea or topic to another. Lack of understanding of behavioural responses to these problems may result in a patient being incorrectly labelled as lacking in motivation and this will result in failure to take the necessary remedial action.

The **environment to which the patient can expect to return**, his **personality, drive, intellectual ability** and **expectations** are all major determinants of outcome as they will influence motivation.[18] The therapist requires an understanding of all these factors for each patient so that the programme which is planned will tap his individual resources and attributes, in other words, take advantage of his strengths and not emphasise or reinforce his weaknesses.

5. **Mental stimulation.** Although many patients eventually return to full mental capacity following stroke, it is certain that not enough time and thought are spent on the retraining of thinking skills. A study done by Kinsella and Ford[33] showed insignificant improvement in intellectual competence in a small group of patients over a period of 12 weeks, although improvement was made on the other measured parameters, such as functional movement. Although, as the authors comment, this result could be attributed to the insensitivity of the tests or the size of the group, it is also probable that, where there are problems of intellect, improvement will not occur without specific training.

For the first few weeks after stroke, many patients describe a feeling of slowness in thinking and a difficulty with concentration. They may be aware of a difficulty with organisation of their thoughts. It has been suggested[34] that brain responses are slowed because of the asynchronous activity of the two hemispheres. Certain factors may accentuate the above problems and should be considered in rehabilitation. The 'isolated' patient, that is, the dysphasic patient, the patient left in bed 'to rest', left to sit alone, or placed beside a television set which he cannot see, begins to experience intellectual regression. Illness and certain drugs can also have a profound effect upon intellectual function and alertness, especially in elderly people.[35] Drowsiness and inability to concentrate may be the result of drug therapy and the rehabilitation team should question the necessity for such medication.

Removal from his habitual environment, particularly in the presence of communication problems, can have a similar effect and the presence of relatives and the organisation of his day to simulate a relatively normal day may therefore make a marked difference to the patient. The rehabilitation team must be careful not to assume that the depressed, labile, confused patient has permanent intellectual impairment, and should set about analysing these problems just as they would analyse the physical problems.

Some patients have problems with memory and with mental functions which may be related to memory. These may be specific and involve an inability to recognise faces, or they may be represented by an inability to remember significant events, dates or places, or an inability to remember motor activities which were practised the previous day. Specific memory training may be helpful for such patients. It is probable, however, that the inability to remember the day-to-day activities of the rehabilitation unit frequently represents the fact that no significant events occurred, that nothing that occurred was actually memorable and that, with no daily timetable or regularity upon which to fix an event, one day has merely merged with the next. More knowledge of how a patient actually spends his day[36] would probably explain his inability to remember.

Old age is sometimes considered to be the reason why a patient is slow to learn. However, a study[37] has shown that both aged and brain-damaged patients appear to have learning potential that does not differ from the younger subjects except for a time factor and a greater need for positive reinforcement. Old age in the chronological sense should not be considered as a barrier to rehabilitation.[11] Gersten[38] reviews some of the literature which examines the relationship between age and outcome of rehabilitation and he concludes that, whatever the relationship, it appears to be mediated by self-concept, family support and social activity.

Early experience of erect positions (sitting and standing) stimulates mental alertness. The MRP provides mental stimulation by demanding the patient's participation and involvement and by its emphasis on the cognitive phase of learning. However, many patients should also participate in a **mental stimulation programme** planned by a neuropsychologist and designed to help the person organise his thinking, and to retrain specifically those cognitive and perceptual abilities he lacks.

6. **Educational programmes.** An education programme for relatives and patients should consist of some lectures and group discussions on the pathophysiology of stroke, the meaning of symptoms, the adaptability of the brain, the physical and emotional effects of stroke, ways of communicating with the person who is dysphasic, planning for discharge, and family and community participation in rehabilitation.

One study[39] to assess the benefit of educational programmes for the patient and his relatives showed support and approval, and another study[40] showed that rehabilitation gains were maintained as well through education of the family as through the use of community services. This latter study also showed an increase, compared with similar studies done in 1958 and 1963, in accepting attitudes of both the rehabilitant and a significant family member. A survey[41] of family members following an educational programme showed decreased anxiety about stroke as well as more effective involvement in the rehabilitation process.[41]

Relatives should be helped to see the significance of their support in helping the patient regain his self-esteem. They will also gain an understanding of the patient's problems through discussion with the rehabilitation staff and by actually participating in treatment sessions. This will motivate them towards carrying out recommendations. If relatives do not know what the patient is accomplishing in therapy, they will expect a lower level of performance at home.[42] They are, if they are educated from the onset of rehabilitation, being prepared for the patient's return home.

Relatives are, in most cases, untapped resources. If the therapist involves them in treatment from the onset, they will be able to give the patient opportunities for practice outside therapy hours. Lack of participation by relatives may result in them being fearful of their ability to cope once the patient goes home. The patient for his part will be motivated by the knowledge that the members of his family feel confident in their role and that he is not necessarily seen by them as a burden. Some suitable publications for patients and their relatives are listed at the end of this section.[26,29,43-45] The list includes articles and books by patients themselves.

An in-service educational programme will enable the physiotherapist to explain how she teaches a patient everyday activities such as standing up and walking. Not everyone will be teaching him these activities but each will need to understand how best to help him to practise. This is particularly important for nursing staff, aides and assistants, who are in constant contact with the patient but whose job should not be to teach him how to move again but to give him the chance to practise correctly. All members of the team need to know how much assistance to give the patient, otherwise he may be left to struggle on his own or he may be given so much help that he is relatively passive. Information should be updated as the patient improves. Other members of the team will thus be able to reinforce throughout the day what the patient is learning and give him the **opportunity to practise, to achieve mastery and to transfer what he has been learning into his everyday activities.** Similarly, the speech pathologist will advise other members of the team on the best ways of communicating with the person who is dysphasic and of reinforcing his attempts to speak.

Educational programmes should also involve sessions aimed at helping staff understand the reasons for various types of behaviour demonstrated by stroke patients and ways of creating the best possible environment for recovery. Isaacs[18] comments that dissemination within the team of practical information about stroke is a most important aspect of rehabilitation. Feigenson[8] adds the point that successful rehabilitation requires organisation within the team, co-ordination of the patient's programmes and the ability to keep everyone inspired.

Two problems which the patient may suffer early after his stroke, and which need particularly to be understood by staff and relatives, are **outbursts of weeping** and **urinary incontinence**.

**Weeping**, which is distressing for patient, relatives and staff, represents a lack of physical as well as emotional control and the patient needs constructive help (see p. 72), a strategy to help him regain control, rather than expressions of sympathy. The therapist who does not understand the reasons for this weeping may make an inappropriate response, suggesting, for example, that treatment be postponed until next day 'when he is feeling better'.

Many patients immediately following stroke experience some urinary and bowel **incontinence**. This is very embarrassing and will increase the person's already high level of anxiety. This state of affairs will be reinforced by constant reference by the staff to his incontinence. Certain factors add to the possibility of having an accident: the person with communication problems will have difficulty making his needs understood; the use of a pan or bottle in bed normally requires use of both hands and reasonable balance and agility, neither of which the patient has.

The patient needs reassurance that he will quickly regain control of bladder and bowel. If he has a communication problem, a way of telling the staff that he wants to go to the lavatory should be established. Staff should ensure that the patient who needs to re-establish control does not have to wait for assistance. He should use a commode rather than a bed pan. Catheterisation should be avoided as it is detrimental to the person's psychological well-being and may provoke urinary tract infection and encourage dependence rather than the gaining of control.

However, the most essential factor in regaining control is the early assumption of the upright position and movement within this position. Standing and moving about in standing will quickly enable the patient to regain control. Incontinence should not be allowed to interfere with or delay treatment, and accidents can be avoided by ensuring that the patient goes to the lavatory before his treatment sessions and at regular intervals throughout the day. Hospital staff should be aware that incontinence is often only a manifestation of the patient's inability to wait or his difficulty communicating his needs. Persistent incontinence should be investigated by a urologist.

7. **Planning for discharge.** Preparation for returning home involves a home visit by a therapist to assess whether or not any adaptation of the house is necessary, and a weekend leave from the rehabilitation unit. Although the authors' clinical experience indicates that the majority of patients do well when rehabilitation is appropriate, some patients will not regain independence, and will require organisation of domiciliary services, such as meals on wheels, home help, or a visiting nurse. The patient with restricted mobility should have access to a list of shops and other buildings free of architectural barriers. An introduction to a Stroke Club,[44] where patients and their relatives can express and share difficulties and experiences and participate in social activities, will help the patient develop social and personal confidence and make easier his return into the community. A member of the rehabilitation team should visit the patient in his home after he has returned home to see if he is maintaining his level of performance, to solve any unforeseen problems and to ensure that the patient is happy and active. Further consultation with a

physiotherapist can be arranged if necessary through the Stroke Club.

## A NOTE ON SENSORY PROBLEMS

Somatosensory and perceptual-motor problems seem to be relatively common immediately following stroke, but with many people they probably, in these early stages, represent a 'confused' state of mind rather than a real deficit. The patient's sensory dysfunction does not arise from problems of a peripheral nature but from difficulty perceiving or interpreting sensory input. The authors' experience with the MRP indicates that the emphasis placed on learning to use and be aware of the affected side and the space it occupies usually corrects these problems and apparently prevents them from becoming established. This may be due to the brain gaining practical experience of monitoring motor performance in conjunction with the therapist's verbal monitoring. Active movement itself may be sufficient sensory stimulus.

Sensory and perceptual problems should not be considered a poor prognostic sign, as a barrier to rehabilitation, or as a reason for failure in rehabilitation, but as factors to be considered in the design of the patient's entire programme. The physiotherapist and neuropsychologist must work actively in training the patient to overcome these deficits just as the physiotherapist will train the patient to overcome his motor deficit.

Much of the literature on sensory and perceptual problems is confusing. Many studies[11, 46–49] concerned with the relationship between sensory dysfunction and prediction of outcome do not indicate whether or not the patients are having any specific training for their deficits. The results of such studies are frequently conflicting. Some authors suggest that proprioceptive dysfunction, for example, affects outcome, others that this is only when it is combined with dysphasia. Other authors consider it does not affect outcome but may affect length of stay. It is difficult to compare these results because of differences in the methods of measuring outcome.

Some of the confusion in terms of perceptual problems arises because they are little understood, are difficult to describe, to categorise and therefore to test. Roy,[50] for example, has pointed out that although many types of apraxia have been described, little is understood about its true nature. Unfortunately, many neuropsychological tests are multifactorial and in many cases the exact nature of the function which is being tested is unknown.[51,52] Furthermore, the patient may improve his performance of the test but may not improve in any functional activity. In addition, there are few normative data on the sensory and motor abilities of the age group which makes up the largest number of stroke patients.[53,54] It needs to be kept in mind that, no matter what tests are devised, the results of assessment are only clinically useful if viewed in terms of providing strategies for remediation.

As has been proposed earlier, many patients immediately following stroke demonstrate what could be called perceptual 'confusion'. For example, they may have some disorder of body image and unilateral spatial neglect. It is as if the person has difficulty organising the material derived from sensory stimuli. He may have a tendency to give up instead of trying to solve the problem or he may make an inappropriate excuse for his difficulty. The MRP, with its emphasis on early weight-bearing through the affected side, training of movement in upright positions, elimination of both unnecessary muscle activity and excessive or unnecessary sensory input to the intact side, patient participation and the use of visual and auditory feedback, appears to prevent the entrenchment of perceptual problems in many patients. Problems may persist, however, in some patients, and a particular deficit will need to be analysed and remediated.

A patient with a perceptual problem is often easily distractable. He may have difficulty shutting out or ignoring extraneous stimuli, noise or bright colours, for example. In this case, he will concentrate better in a quiet room without distractions. Sensory bombardment (by brushing, icing, vibration or towelling), which is sometimes suggested as a means of improving the patient's awareness of his affected side, may increase his confusion, giving him a variety of inputs when he is unable to cope with all the information he is already receiving. Furthermore, McMahon[55] suggests that where vibration is given as part of a generalised sensory regime to increase awareness and responsiveness, it may actually minimise or even prevent the awareness of all subsequent inputs. This illustrates the inappropriateness of arbitrary, non-specific sensory stimulation programmes.

**Astereognosis** and poor **two-point discrimination**, if they persist, will interfere in particular with hand function and may need to be improved by direct practice.[56–58]

If **tactile or visual inattention** (extinction) is present, all stimuli to the intact side should be reduced and stimuli given only to the affected side, with cognitive awareness of the stimulus encouraged. Gradually, the patient is taught to cope with conflicting stimuli to both sides of the body without extinguishing the stimulus to the affected side.

Patients with **visual field defects**, such as homonymous hemianopia, may need to be trained to turn the head to compensate for lack of vision, but it may be possible to train vision within the area of deficits.

**Unilateral spatial neglect**, which may be a persistent problem in some patients, is considered to be accompanied by a shift to one side of the subjective midpoint of the body.[59] Hence the patient tends, visually and physically, to drift towards one side. In therapy, he is made aware of the problem and given a solution. He is constantly reminded of how to regain his body alignment by consciously shifting his weight on to his affected leg and of the need to stay there. A limb load monitor* will help him by providing an auditory reminder of the position of his centre of gravity. He is helped to learn again where the real midline of his body is by using weight-bearing through the affected leg as one anchor and vision as another. Weight-bearing through the affected leg is encouraged if he wears a calico splint (p. 108) to support his knee.

His vision is directed towards his affected side. He is encouraged to

*Krusen Research Center, Philadelphia, Pennsylvania.

search for a particular object. The therapist should get eye contact and 'draw' his attention towards his affected side by getting him to maintain eye contact as he moves his head. Whenever his weight or his gaze drifts back to his intact side, he needs verbal feedback and manual or visual guidance to remind him to use these two anchors. It is worth noting that the patient who drifts to one side does badly if he is held up by the therapist, or is pushed or pulled towards the affected side. The therapist should therefore give only the minimum amount of physical support and guidance.

From the onset of rehabilitation, the therapist must be careful not to reinforce this neglect. If the patient persists, for example, in looking always to one side, the therapist will have to avoid consciously a natural tendency to fit in with this behaviour. She must constantly draw his attention and his gaze towards the affected side by speaking to him from this side, by encouraging weight-bearing through this side and by instructing other staff in the need to be consistent in this matter. Standing up by pivoting on the intact leg will reinforce a unilateral neglect and will encourage him not to use the affected side (see Fig. 6.10).

Specific training may be necessary for some patients. Weinberg and Diller and their co-workers[60] describe a study in which an experimental group of patients with unilateral spatial neglect was given specific training in visual scanning. In a later study,[61] another experimental group of patients was given training in sensory awareness and spatial re-organisation. Both studies indicated that these patients showed superior performance in the retest compared to the control group which was having 'traditional' rehabilitation. Diller[62] and his colleagues are at present continuing with a study of the effect of a spatial awareness programme upon people with spatial neglect.

**Vision** can be said to have two objectives in respect to movement: the location of objects in space, and orientation of the body in space.[63] The former enables accurate goal-directed motor actions. The latter involves the postural adjustments necessary for particular movements to take place and probably affects motoneuron excitability in the muscles which are responsible for the movement.[63,64]

A person who is having difficulty with head and trunk control in the sitting position in the first few days following stroke may actually be having difficulty with visual control. If he finds it difficult to look at the therapist's face or at his own hand when attempting arm movement, he may be having difficulty locating what he must look at. Normally, when a person needs to locate visually an object within the peripheral visual field, there need to be saccadic eye movements and head movements which enable the object to be imaged by the fovea, which is the most sensitive part of the retina. The central nervous system needs to process the information it receives in order to produce co-ordination between eye and head movement. The therapist needs to consider the relationship between eye movement, head movement and postural adjustment, for example, by giving the patient practice in searching for (i.e. locating) and fixating on particular objects.

Many stroke patients would normally wear glasses to correct visual dysfunction, particularly when using the hands for fine motor skills, and the therapist should ensure that such a person wears his glasses during therapy.[65] It also needs to be remembered that older people may have decreased visual acuity because of cataract, glaucoma or senile macular degeneration.

Therapists should question existing ways of looking at sensory and perceptual problems and work with neuropsychologists to explore new ideas of remediation. Isaacs[66] reports a suggestion by W. M. R. McLean, for example, that neglect of the left half of space may be due to overactivity of the intact hemisphere, that is, to suppression of the affected side by visual input from the normal side. The suggested treatment, which is under further study, is to obscure the right visual field with special spectacles.

Below is a summary of the major factors in creating the right environment for the stroke patient.

1. If the patient is to make his best possible recovery from the effects of stroke, he must be in an environment in which he can receive effective diagnostic and medical care, an environment which reduces the likelihood of complications, motivates him and encourages him to learn. The advantage of a specialised stroke unit is that all staff are trained to bring this situation about. It is unfortunate that, at present, most medical and therapy personnel consider themselves equipped for stroke care. This is not so and serves to illustrate the lack of understanding, prevalent in the health professions, of the adaptability of the brain and, hence, of the need for specialised rehabilitation.

2. Rehabilitation must commence within the first few days after stroke in order to prevent learned non-use of the affected side, and mental and perceptual-motor deterioration, and to stimulate the patient's learning abilities in both motor and mental function.

3. Rehabilitation should consist of programmes specific to each patient's problems, and should include not only a motor programme, but also programmes designed to overcome his specific perceptual-motor, visual, mental and speech problems. The patient's day must be planned in such a way that he is taught and given practice in leading a 'normal' day, learning to take responsibility, to regain a sense of time, etc. No part of his day should be spent on activities irrelevant to normal life.

4. If the patient is to be motivated to regain a normal capacity for life, such motivation must be planned and not left to the discretion of individual therapists.

5. Consistency between the activities the patient learns with the therapist and performance of these activities with other members of the staff during the day must be ensured. Furthermore, just as the patient expects to be treated by the same physician while he requires medical care, so also should he have the right to the same therapist throughout his rehabilitation.

## REFERENCES

1. WHO (1971). Cerebrovascular disease: prevention, treatment and re-

habilitation. *Wld Hlth Org. techn. Rep. Ser*; 469

2. Langton Hewer R. (1976). Stroke rehabilitation. In *Stroke* (Gillingham F. J., Mawdsley C., and Williams A. E. eds.) pp. 476–490. London: Churchill Livingstone.

3. Steers A. J. W. (1976). Immediate care of stroke. In *Stroke* (Gillingham F. J., Mawdsley C., and Williams A. E. eds) pp. 263–273. London: Churchill Livingstone.

4. United States Department of Health Education and Welfare (1976). *Guidelines for Stroke Care*. Washington DC: United States Government Printing Office.

5. Weisberg L. A. and Nice C. N. (1977). Intracranial tumors simulating the presentation of cerebrovascular symptoms. Early detection with cerebral computed tomography (CCT). *Amer. J. Med*; **63**:517.

6. Brocklehurst J. C., Andrews K., Morris P. E., Richards B. R. and Laycock P. L. (1978). Why admit patients to hospital? *Age and Ageing*; **7**:100–108.

7. Mulley G. and Aire T. (1978). Treating stroke: home or hospital. *Brit. med. J*; **2**:1321.

8. Feigenson J. S. (1979). Editorial. Stroke rehabilitation: effectiveness, benefit and costs. Some practical considerations. *Stroke*; **10**:1–4.

9. Kottke F. J. (1974). Historia obscura hemiplegiae. *Arch. phys. Med*; **55**:4–13.

10. Lehmann J. F., De Lateur B. J., Fowler R. S. *et al.* (1975). Stroke: does rehabilitation effect outcome? *Arch. phys. Med*; **56**:375–82.

11. Feigenson J. S., McDowell F. H., Meese P., McCarthy M. L. and Greenberg S. D. (1977). Factors influencing outcome and length of stay in a stroke rehabilitation unit. Part 1. *Stroke*; **8**:651–6.

12. Drake W. E., Hamilton M. J., Carlsson M. and Blumenkrantz J. (1973). Acute stroke management and patient outcome: the value of neurovascular care units. *Stroke*; **4**:933–45.

13. McCann B. C. and Culbertson R. A. (1976). Comparisons of 2 systems for stroke rehabilitation in a general hospital. *J. Amer. Geriat. Soc*; **24**:211–216.

14. Isaacs B. (1976). The place of a stroke unit in geriatric medicine. *Physiotherapy*; **62**:152–4.

15. Feigenson J. S. and McCarthy M. L. (1977). Guidelines for establishing a stroke rehabilitation unit. *N. Y. St. J. Med*; August:1430–34.

16. Howard B. E. (1977). A Practical Approach to Care of the Acute Stroke Patient in a Community Hospital Setting. Unpublished paper given at the *53rd National Congress of APTA, St. Louis, Missouri*.

17. Garraway W. M., Akhtar A. J., Prescott R. J. and Hockey L. (1980). Management of acute stroke in the elderly: preliminary results of a controlled trial. *Brit. med. J*; 12 April: 1040–43.

18. Isaacs B. (1978). Stroke. Who cares? In *Textbook of Geriatric Medicine and Gerontology*, 2nd edn. (Brocklehurst J. C. ed.) pp. 201–220. London: Churchill Livingstone.

19. Feigenson J. S., Gitlow H. S. and Greenberg S. D. (1979). Disability oriented rehabilitation unit—a major factor influencing stroke outcome. *Stroke*; **10**:5–8.

20. Stern P. H., McDowell F., Miller J. M. and Robinson M. (1971). Factors influencing stroke rehabilitation. *Stroke*; **2**:213.

21. Anderson T. P., Bourestom N., Greenberg F. R. and Hildyard V. G. (1974). Predictive factors in stroke rehabilitation. *Arch. phys. Med*; **55**:545–53.

22. Robinson R. A. (1976). Psychiatric aspects of stroke. In *Stroke* (Gillingham C., Mawdsley C. and Williams A. E., eds.) pp. 490–504. London: Churchill Livingstone.

23. Bexton W. H., Heron W. and Scott T. H. (1956). Effects of decreased

variation in the sensory environment. *Canadian J. Psychol*; **8**:70–76.

24. Walsh R. and Greenough W., eds. (1976). *Environments as Therapy for Brain Dysfunction*. New York: Plenum Press.

25. Seligman M. (1975). In *Helplessness on Depression, Development and Death*. pp. 21–41, 180–188. San Francisco: W. H. Freeman.

26. Griffiths V. (1970). *A Stroke in the Family*. London: Pitman.

27. Rosenzweig M. R., Bennett E. L. and Diamond M. C. (1967). Effects of differential environment on brain anatomy and brain chemistry. *Proc. Amer. psychopath. Ass*; **56**:45–6.

28. Walsh R. N. (1981). Sensory environments, brain damage and drugs: A review of interactions and mediating mechanisms. *Int. J. Neuroscience*; **14**:129–37.

29. Hodgins E. (1966). Listen: the patient. *New Engl. J. Med*; **274**:657–61.

30. Belmont I., Benjamin H., Ambrose J. and Restuccia R. D. (1969). Effect of cerebral damage on motivation in rehabilitation. *Arch. phys. Med*; **50**:507–11.

31. Kottke F. J. (1975). Neurophysiologic therapy for stroke. In *Stroke and its Rehabilitation* (Licht S., ed.) pp. 255–324. New Haven: Elizabeth Licht.

32. Hyman M. D. (1972). Social isolation and performance, *J. chron. Dis*; **25**:85–97.

33. Kinsella G. and Ford B. (1980). Acute recovery pattern in stroke patients. *Med. J. Aust*; 13 December: 653–66.

34. Belmont I., Karp E. and Birch H. G. (1971). Hemispheric inco-ordination in hemiplegia. *Brain*; **94**:337–48.

35. Linford Rees W. (1979). Rehabilitation in the elderly. *Biblthca Psychiat*; **159**:155–62.

36. Keith R. A. and Sharp K. W. (1980). Time use of stroke patients in three rehabilitation hospitals. *Arch phys. Med*; **61**:501–503.

37. Halberstam J. L. and Zaretsky H. H. (1969). Learning capacities of the elderly and brain-damaged. *Arch. phys. Med*; **50**:133–9.

38. Gersten J. W. (1975). Rehabilitation potential. In *Stroke and its Rehabilitation* (Licht S. ed.) pp. 435–471. New Haven: Elizabeth Licht.

39. Medcalf T. E. and Vandiver R. L. (1980). Stroke forum. *Phys. Ther*; **60**:905.

40. Anderson E., Anderson T. P. and Kottke F. J. (1977). Stroke rehabilitation: maintenance of achieved gains. *Arch phys. Med*; **58**:345–52.

41. Wells R. (1974). Family stroke education. *Stroke*; **5**:393–6.

42. Andrews K. and Stewart J. (1979). Stroke recovery: he can but does he? *Rheumatology and Rehabilitation*; **18**:43–8.

43. Carr J. H. and Shepherd R. B. (1979). *Early Care of the Stroke Patient. A Positive Approach*. London: Heinemann Medical.

44. Griffiths V. (1978). *Volunteer Stroke Scheme Handbook*. London: Chest, Heart and Stroke Association.

45. Saw R. (1981). *The One-fingered Typist*. Sydney: Wildcat Press.

46. Hurwitz L. J. and Adams G. F. (1972). Rehabilitation of hemiplegia: indices of assessment and prognosis. *Brit. med. J*; 8 January: 94–8.

47. Isaacs B. and Mark R. (1973). Determinants of outcome of stroke rehabilitation. *Age and Ageing*; **2**:139–49.

48. Feigenson J. S., McCarthy M. L., Greenberg S. D. and Feigenson W. D. (1977). Factors influencing outcome and length of stay in a stroke rehabilitation unit. Part 2. *Stroke*; **8**:657–62.

49. McClatchie G. (1980). Survey of rehabilitation outcome of strokes. *Med. J. Aust*; June 28: 649–51.

50. Roy E. A. (1978). Apraxia: a new look at an old syndrome. *J. Human Movt. Studies*; **4**:191–210.

51. Walsh K. (1978). *Neuropyschology and Clinical Approach*. London: Churchill Livingstone.
52. Siev E. and Freishtat B. (1976). *Perceptual Dysfunction in the Adult Stroke Patient*. New Jersey: Charles B. Slack.
53. Welford A. T. (1959). Psychomotor performance. In *Handbook of Aging and the Individual* (Birren J. E. ed.) pp. 562–614. Chicago: University of Chicago Press.
54. Woodburn L. S. (1967). Partial analysis of the neural elements in posture and locomotion. *Psychol. Bull*; **68**:121–48.
55. McMahon C. (1981). Rationale for the use of vibration in the management of tactile defensive patients. *Aust. J. Physiother*; **27**:75–9.
56. Carr J. and Shepherd R. (1980). *Physiotherapy in Disorders of the Brain*. London: Heinemann Medical.
57. Abercrombie M. L. J. (1968). Some notes on spatial disability: movement, intelligence quotient and attentiveness. *Develop. Med. Child Neurol*; **10**:206–13.
58. Inglis J., Sproule M., Leicht M., Donald M. W. and Campbell D. (1976). Electromyographic biofeedback treatment of residual neuromuscular disabilities after cerebrovascular accident. *Physiotherapy Canada*; **28**:260–64.
59. Apfeldorf M. (1962). Perceptual and conceptual processes in case of left-sided spatial inattention. *Percept. Motor Skills*; **14**:419–23.
60. Weinberg J., Diller L., Gordon W., Gerstman L. J., Lieberman A., Lakin P., Hodges G. and Ezrachi O. (1977). Visual scanning training effect on reading-related tasks in acquired right brain damage. *Arch. phys. Med*; **58**:479–86.
61. Weinberg J., Diller L., Gordon W., Gerstman L. J., Lieberman A., Lakin P., Hodges G. and Ezrachi O. (1979). Training sensory awareness and spatial organisation in people with right brain damage. *Arch. phys. Med*; **60**:491–6.
62. Diller L. (1981). Personal communication.
63. Herman R., Herman R. and Maulucci R. (1981). Visually triggered eye–arm movements in man. *Exp. Brain Res*; **42**:392–8.
64. Herman R., Cook T., Cozzins B. and Freedman W. (1974). Control of postural reactions in man: the initiation of gait. In *Control of Posture and Locomotion* (Stein R. B., Pearson K. G., Smith R. S. and Redford J. B. eds.) pp. 363–88. New York: Plenum Press.
65. Macfarlane A. and Longhurst E. C. (1979–80). Visual assessment of cerebrovascular accident patients in rehabilitation programmes. *Australian Orthoptic Journal*; **17**:42–7.
66. Isaacs B. (1977). Stroke research and the physiotherapist. *Physiotherapy*; **63**:366–8.

# PART II

# The Motor Relearning Programme

# 1

# *Introduction*

The MRP is made up of seven sections representing the essential functions of everyday life: upper limb function, oro-facial function, sitting up from supine, sitting, standing up and sitting down, standing, and walking. The first two sections comprise activities grouped together for ease of reference.

Within each section is a prescribed plan of action, laid out in four steps (Table 1.1) and preceded by a description of the normal activity, including the most essential movement components.

The order in which the sections appear is unimportant as there is no intent of progression from section to section. The therapist may start a treatment session with whatever section or part of a section is most appropriate for the patient. It is not necessary for a patient to perfect a part of a section before going on to another section. Each treatment session should comprise material from all sections.

The MRP should commence as soon as the patient is medically stable. Should he be confined to bed for a short period following his stroke, he should start on the parts of the Programme which he can manage, for example, oro-facial function, upper limb function and extension of the hip in preparation for standing.

The MRP is intended to be sufficient in itself as a programme for the regaining of movement and motor control following stroke. The addition of conflicting techniques will interfere with the training process.

However, methods of stimulating specific muscle action or movement components, which also provide auditory or visual evidence of muscle contraction (for example, biofeedback[1,2] or mechanical vibration[3-5]) may be introduced since they do not conflict with the principles underlying the Programme. Similarly, information from research into studies of hemispheric specialisation and hemispheric interference, for example, may enable the methods of training motor control to become more specific than they are at present. More recent studies of brain function have considered the complex interactions between the two cerebral hemispheres,[6] whereas previously, the right hemisphere was considered the 'minor' hemisphere, and there was a simplistic view of dominance which inferred that one hemisphere was totally dominant. It is now understood that each hemisphere has specialised functions and that the two

27

**Table 1.1** *The four steps in the Motor Relearning Programme*

| | |
|---|---|
| **Step 1** | **Analysis of function** |
| | Observation |
| | Comparison |
| | Analysis |
| | |
| **Step 2** | **Practice of missing components** |
| | Explanation + instructions |
| | Practice (with verbal feedback + |
| | manual guidance) |
| | |
| **Step 3** | **Practice of activity** |
| | Explanation + instructions |
| | Practice (with verbal feedback + |
| | manual guidance) |
| | Progression: |
| |    increase complexity |
| |    add variety |
| |    decrease feedback + guidance |
| | |
| **Step 4** | **Transference of learning** |
| | Opportunity to practise |
| | Consistency of practice |
| | Involvement of relatives and staff |
| | Positive reinforcement |
| | Stimulating environment |

hemispheres work together to complement each other. The term 'dominance' is now used to relate to a particular modality. For example, the right hemisphere is considered to be dominant in terms of visuospatial functioning.

An understanding of the functions in which each hemisphere is dominant and of the way in which the hemispheres interact and complement each other in the organisation of behaviour will enable the therapist to determine, in training motor control, those modalities upon which she should concentrate with a particular patient. Certainly, in administering this Programme, the therapist should consider switching from verbal instruction to visual demonstration or *vice versa* if a person does not respond.

The various sections of the Programme will make up the patient's daily therapy sessions, which should range from at least half an hour twice daily in the first few days to daily one-hour sessions or preferably more. The activities the patient has been practising will need to be reinforced outside therapy sessions, and relatives and staff should be encouraged to participate and trained to be consistent. A particular routine or 'drill', carried over from therapy sessions into the rest of the patient's day, is essential for consistency of performance and the learning of motor control. The plan of action is outlined in four steps (Table 1.1).

**Step 1** involves recognition and analysis of each problem. This enables the correct decisions to be made about treatment.

The therapist **observes** the patient as he performs or attempts to perform an activity, for example standing up.

She **analyses** the movement and **notes** the missing components, the absence of muscle activity and the presence of any excessive or inappropriate muscle activity.

In analysing the activity, she **asks questions** about the patient's behaviour. For example, 'Why does his knee hyperextend when he takes weight through it?' The therapist must ask herself whether his problem is due to lack of control of the quadriceps in 0–15° of extension. Is this lack of control associated with unnecessary muscle activity, such as hyperactivity of the plantarflexors? Is his knee position due to abnormal hip alignment (i.e. flexed instead of extended) or due to his knee being pushed back into extension passively by the therapist as she helps him stand up (see Fig. 6.7). She must differentiate between primary problems and those which are merely secondary in order to make the correct decision about the problems to which treatment must be directed.

It is only by making a thorough analysis of each motor problem, which includes any anatomical, biomechanical, physiological and behavioural factors, that the therapist will be able to make the correct decisions about treatment and examples of the influence of these factors are given throughout the text. The degree to which the therapist understands the muscle activity and movements involved in everyday activities, and her knowledge of the factors underlying the patient's problems will determine the accuracy of both her analysis of movement and her selection of components on which to concentrate.

In Step 1 there is a guide to the most commonly missing components and the ways in which a patient may compensate. Having decided on the movement components which are missing, the therapist, using the description of the normal movement as a guide, selects those which are essential to the activity, that is, those which are the determinants, the biomechanical necessities, upon which the activity depends. It is these components upon which the therapist and patient will concentrate in treatment. For example, if a patient can barely move his hand, it is obvious that he is missing many movement components. However, the therapist will select the components most essential to hand use on which to concentrate in treatment (see p. 37). These, once the patient regains some control over them, will act as triggers to the other components which make up particular activities, as they are the components most likely to generalise into many different activities.

Step 1 is continuous throughout **Steps 2 and 3** of the Programme, as the therapist is continually analysing and re-evaluating the patient's responses and the reasons for success or failure, in order to make decisions about the next step in treatment or the next instruction to give. Quick and continuous analysis and decision-making are interwoven throughout the therapy session and dictate the action taken.

This continuous re-evaluation also provides feedback to the therapist about the effectiveness of analysis and decision-making as well as of treatment. If the patient's performance is not successful, the therapist needs to check her original analysis of his problems as well as consider whether or not the technique was properly carried out. Errors in analysis are frequently the cause of ineffective treatment. Evaluation is, of course, closely linked to expectation. For the therapist to see the need for an immediate re-evaluation of her analysis of a particular problem she must have an expectation of success; that is, she must start the treatment session expecting the patient to show improvement in everything he practises throughout that session.

Although Steps 2 and 3 overlap, Step 2 is the practice of a component, a 'warm-up' which prepares the patient for performancě of the entire skill in Step 3. Step 2 should stimulate mental as well as physical 'readiness'. Monitoring and training of balanced alignment will be interspersed throughout the Programme. All activities in which the body is affected by gravity require continuous balance adjustments.

There are three important points to be considered.

1. **Activities or motor tasks are either practised in their entirety or they are broken down into their components**, practice of each component being followed immediately by practice of the entire activity. Many patients in the early stages will be unable to practise the entire activity, and will have to practise each movement component, with emphasis frequently on the stimulation of individual muscles. The patient must understand what he is preparing for, and this preparation must be immediately followed by performance of at least part of the activity for which he is preparing. For example, he may practise controlling his quadriceps in sitting (p. 127), in preparation for controlling flexion–extension of the knee through stance phase of walking. He should then stand up and practise weight-bearing through the leg and taking a step forward with the intact leg, although he may not be able to walk that day. By practising in this way he will be able to see where the muscle activity or component fits in to the sequence of the entire activity.

However, in some cases, practice of the entire activity with manual guidance from the therapist to ensure normal speed, rhythm, timing and sequencing will actually trigger off the memory of the movements required, even if at first the patient makes some errors. The negative effect of the errors may be unimportant compared with the positive effect of the rhythm of the activity. Once the patient has the 'idea' of the movement, he can go back to practise particular components in order to become more skilled.

2. **Techniques** principally comprise verbal and visual feedback and instruction and manual guidance. Before he begins to practise, the patient receives an **explanation** and a **demonstration** to help him understand the reason he is having difficulty, that is, the necessity of the component on

which he will concentrate and practise. Sometimes this is sufficient to trigger the patient's memory for the movement and he can go on to practise the entire activity immediately without having to practise the component separately.

Brief **instructions** are given as a guide to the points which should be emphasised to the patient, and also because an appropriate verbal cue is an important technique for triggering off movement. These instructions may need to be replaced or reinforced by non-verbal communication, such as gestures and demonstrations, if the patient has difficulty in synthesising this information, for example if he is dysphasic. **Verbal feedback**, also brief, relevant and concise, is continuous throughout treatment, being given both during the performance and at its end. **Manual guidance**, in terms of a physical monitoring of the patient's performance to ensure correct alignment and to guide the movement, is also continuous throughout the performance. Although the therapist may move the patient passively in order to show him what he must practise, she should be careful not to persist with passive movements beyond one or two demonstrations. She should give him the opportunity to attempt an active movement, monitor his attempts verbally, and manually guide him so he performs at least part of the movement actively.

**Points to check** have been suggested in Steps 2 and 3 in order to indicate errors which are commonly made either by the therapist or by the patient and which will certainly interfere with performance. The commonest error is a failure to monitor body alignment. This monitoring is essential throughout the therapy session as normal alignment will ensure that the appropriate muscles are placed at a mechanical advantage for the action required.

3. **Methods of progression**. It is important that the patient practises at peak performance, his abilities continually being progressed to their limits. Furthermore, he should not waste time by practising what he can already do. Activities are progressed as soon as he has some control. Movements are made more complex by a decrease in manual guidance and feedback, by alterations in speed, and by adding variety. As the patient regains some skill in an activity, he should be exposed to different situations in order to improve his performance and to enable him to react favourably to the unexpected. During Step 3, as he develops skill, the patient makes the transition from the cognitive phase of learning to the automatic phase of learning.

Many of the methods of progression commonly described in the literature on therapy for stroke[7–9] are not appropriate for stroke patients and illustrate a confusion about the meaning of progression. Inappropriate methods of progression include progressing from passive range of motion exercises to resisted exercises, from parallel bars to four-point cane, from a wide base to a narrow base. Other misconceived methods of progression include ensuring that the patient can roll over before he practises balancing in sitting, can crawl before he can walk, can sit on the floor before he can sit on a stool, can move his shoulder before he can move his hand. These ideas originate from the unfortunate and unsubstantiated theory that the adult brain-damaged person regresses to the state of motor immaturity seen in infancy, and hence should be trained to perform motor acts in a so-called neurodevelopmental sequence. These methods of 'progression' are based on false assumptions about normal function, and will prevent the patient from relearning motor control.

**Step 4** describes some ways of ensuring a carry-over of what the patient has been learning in therapy sessions into the rest of his day. This enables him to practise, it gives consistency to his experience and promotes transference of learning. If the patient has been really involved in working out solutions to his problems with his therapist, he will start to apply the same strategies when he is practising on his own. Step 4 is essential because, although the patient may be able to perform a particular component or activity correctly with the therapist, for him to **learn** this component or activity, he will need to practise at other times during the day. As well as having the opportunity to practise physically, he should also spend time practising mentally.

## EQUIPMENT

Very little equipment is necessary for this Programme—a low bed which is of convenient height for the patient to practise standing up and sitting down, several small steps for techniques described in the Programme and for enabling different sized people to sit with feet supported, common objects for retraining hand function and calico splints.

Much physiotherapy equipment traditionally used in stroke re-habilitation is in direct conflict with the principles of the Programme. For example, parallel bars encourage the use of the arms (usually only the intact arm) for weight-bearing, interfere with the relearning of normal body alignment and prevent the trunk from being supported in a balanced manner on both legs. Use of a three- or four-point cane has a similar effect. Some patients may, however, need a regular cane to steady them and some may have used a cane before their stroke. The therapist should ensure that the patient understands that he should not lean on the cane but should use it merely for steadying himself. A longer than normal cane may ensure this.

The use of a device to hold the foot in dorsiflexion (splint, short leg brace with ankle stops) should be avoided. It holds the foot in dorsiflexion throughout the walking cycle, preventing the plantarflexion which is necessary at certain stages of the cycle. The patient will have to compensate by hyperextending his knee or by holding it in flexion during the stance phase.

## SPASTICITY

Throughout the MRP, no direct reference has been made to spasticity. However, in the authors' opinion, what is usually called spasticity is, in most patients following stroke unnecessary muscular activity which has become habitual (see p. 383), certain muscles, those whose mechanical advantage is greatest, contracting persistently to the disadvantage of others. Most patients who commence the MRP immediately following their stroke should not develop disabling muscle imbalance. However, even if a patient starts the Programme when this has already developed, treatment will still consist of the elicitation of appropriate muscle activity and the elimination of unnecessary muscle activity. The objective of treatment, that is, the retraining of motor control, remains the same. An example may make this point clear.

A patient in standing cannot extend his hip to assume the correct standing alignment and his knee is hyperextended. The therapist points out this malalignment to him and asks him to bring his hips forward. He cannot do this and the therapist notes that excessive activity of his ankle plantarflexors is actually pushing his centre of gravity backwards. The objective at this point is to stimulate hip extension while at the same time eliminating excessive activity in the knee extensors and in the ankle plantarflexors. The method described on p. 106 for stimulating hip extension will, with a change in emphasis, achieve this objective.* Initially, the therapist's and patient's attention, however, will have to be more on eliminating knee extension and ankle plantarflexion than on contracting the hip extensors. The flexed knee position (with the knee at a right-angle) will make it easier for the patient to eliminate knee extensor activity perhaps because the quadriceps is prevented from contracting excessively in this position. The therapist, by pushing down firmly through his knee to keep his foot plantigrade, and by holding the toes in dorsiflexion (to prevent toe flexion), helps the patient control the overactivity of the plantarflexors. The manual control plus verbal monitoring of his muscle activity enables him to activate his hip extensors. He then stands up and practises controlling his hip in extension, stepping forward with the intact leg to ensure weight-bearing through the affected leg with the hip in correct alignment. He still attempts cognitively to keep muscle activity at an appropriate level, but the therapist may assist him by holding his toes in dorsiflexion during weight-bearing and by reminding him to extend his hip.

The reader should refer to the Appendices in order to have a better understanding of the way in which the Programme should be used.

## REFERENCES

1. Brudny J., Korein J., Grynbaum B. and Sachs-Frankel G. (1977). Sensory feedback therapy in patients with brain insult. *Scand. J. Rehab. Med*; 9:155–63.
2. Gonella C., Kolish R. and Hole G. (1978). A commentary on electromyographic feedback in physical therapy. *Phys. Ther*; 58:11–14.

*The Bobaths developed a method of decreasing excessive motor activity which they call reflex inhibiting movements.[11] There have been several attempts at explaining their effectiveness, which may, to some extent, be due to the overactive (spastic) muscles being put at a relative disadvantage and the muscles required to contract at a relative advantage.

3. Bishop B. (1975). Vibratory stimulation. Part 3: Possible applications of vibration in treatment of motor dysfunctions. *Phys. Ther*; **55**,2:139–43.
4. Goldfinger G. and Schoon C. (1978). Reliability of the T.V.R. *Phys. Ther*; **58**,1:46–50.
5. McMahon C. (1981). Rationale for the use of vibration in management of tactile defensive patients. *Aust. J. Physiother*; **27**,3:75–9.
6. Stockmeyer S. (1980). Hemispheric Specialisation—General Aspects of Importance to Therapists. Unpublished paper given at the *First Austral-Asian Physiotherapy Congress, Singapore.*
7. Rehabilitation Study Group (1972). 11 Stroke Rehabilitation. *Stroke*; **3**:381.
8. Licht S. (1975). Stroke rehabilitation program. In *Stroke and its Rehabilitation* (Licht S. ed.) pp. 206–220. New Haven: Elizabeth Licht.
9. Johnstone M. (1978). In *Restoration of Motor Function in the Stroke Patient*, pp. 35, 157. London: Churchill Livingstone.
10. Bobath B. (1978). *Adult Hemiplegia* 2nd edn. London: Heinemann Medical.

# 2

# *Upper limb function*

## DESCRIPTION OF NORMAL FUNCTION

Most daily activities involve complex movements of the upper limb. Such activities involve the ability to:

- grasp and release different objects, of different shapes, sizes, weights, textures

- grasp and release different objects with the arm in different relationships to the body (i.e. close to the body, away from the body)

- hold an object while moving the arm (Fig. 2.1)

- move an object about within the hand

- manipulate tools for specific purposes

- reach in all directions (in front, behind, above the head, etc.)

- use two hands together, for example one hand holding and the other moving (Fig. 2.2), both hands doing the same movement (rolling out pastry), both hands doing different movements (piano playing).

There are certain pre-requisites for effective use of the upper limb. These are (i) the ability to look at what one is doing, (ii) the ability to make the postural adjustments which occur with arm movement and which free the hands for manipulation, and (iii) sensory discrimination.

**Fig. 2.1** *Note that the posture of the hand in frame 1 is already appropriate for grasping the glass.*

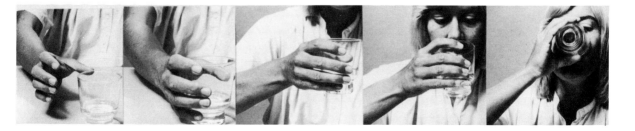

35

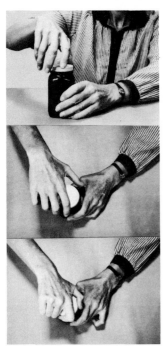

**Fig. 2.2** *Putting the lid on a jar. Note the changing relationship between the hands in frames 2 and 3.*

**Fig. 2.3** *This subject illustrates the arm and body movements involved in reaching down to pick up a cup.*

Sensory discrimination involves the ability to feel an object in the hand, to recognise its nature (that is, its size, shape, form in three dimensions, composition and texture) and the position of the object in the hand. In addition it involves awareness of the relationship of parts of the hand to each other and their position in space. An important aspect of sensory discrimination involves the appreciation of the compressibility of an object, which can be said to involve a combination of dynamaesthesia (the appreciation of the force applied in a motor act), kinaesthesia (the appreciation of change in position of fingers) and the appreciation of counter-pressure of the fingertips.[1]

## ESSENTIAL COMPONENTS

Despite the complexity of upper limb function it is possible to identify the most essential movement components, that is, those components which, when mastered, will allow the performance of many different activities. Performance of these components enables the various parts of the upper limb to assume their optimum postures for function.

### Arm

The major function of the arm is to enable the hand to be positioned for manipulation (Fig. 2.3). Hence the essential components are:

- shoulder abduction
- shoulder forward flexion
- elbow flexion and extension.

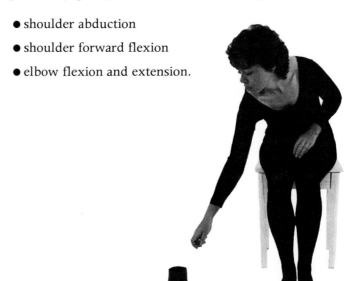

Fig. 2.3

These components are always accompanied by appropriate shoulder girdle movement and rotation at the gleno-humeral joint. It should be noted that the ratio of gleno-humeral to scapulo-thoracic movement is 5:4 after the arm has reached 30° of abduction. Before 30° the ratio is approximately 6:1.

# Hand

The major function of the hand is to grasp, release and manipulate objects. Hence the essential components are:

- radial deviation combined with wrist extension (Fig. 2.4)

- wrist extension while holding an object

- palmar abduction and rotation (opposition) at the carpo-metacarpal joint of the thumb (Fig. 2.5)

- flexion and conjunct rotation (opposition) of individual fingers towards the thumb (Fig. 2.6)

- extension of the metacarpo-phalangeal joints of the fingers with interphalangeal joints in some flexion

- supination of the forearm while holding an object.

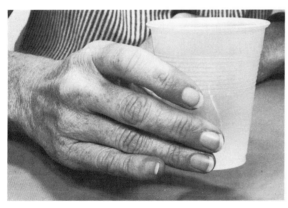

Fig. 2.4

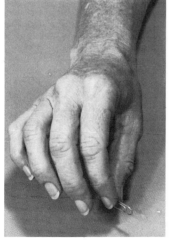

Fig. 2.5

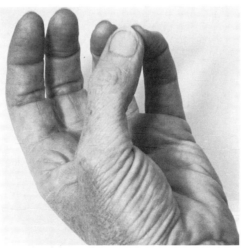

Fig. 2.6

*Fig. 2.4 Radial deviation, wrist extension and finger flexion are essential components ensuring the optimum posturing of the hand for grasp of different objects for different purposes.* **Fig. 2.5** *Combined palmar abduction and rotation at the carpo-metacarpal joint is an essential component for optimum posturing of the thumb for manipulation.* **Fig. 2.6** *The 'cupping' posture of the hand, illustrated here as the subject touches the thumb to little finger, results from flexion of the finger with conjunct rotation towards the thumb.*

## STEP 1    ANALYSIS OF UPPER LIMB FUNCTION

Immediately following stroke, many patients have no easily observable motor activity in the upper limb. However, recovering motor activity *can* be found if the therapist understands muscle function well enough to be able to **search actively** for and **detect** small amounts of muscle activity as soon as they occur. A muscle which may appear non-functioning may contract if the conditions are right. Analysis of muscle activity around the **shoulder** should be done with the patient in **supine** (see Fig. 2.11) until he can control his shoulder in sitting without compensatory movements. Muscle activity in the **hand** is analysed in a similar way but with the **patient sitting at a table**.

Specific problems which may be evident include absence of the essential components plus certain errors of function which illustrate lack of motor control, some muscles demonstrating depressed activity and others excessive and unnecessary activity. The most common problems are the following.

### Arm

- Poor scapular movement (particularly lateral rotation and protraction) and persistent depression of the shoulder girdle.

- Poor muscular control of gleno-humeral joint, that is, lack of shoulder abduction and forward flexion, or inability to sustain these positions. The patient may compensate by using excessive shoulder girdle elevation and lateral flexion of the trunk (Fig. 2.7).

- Excessive and unnecessary elbow flexion, internal rotation of shoulder and pronation of forearm.

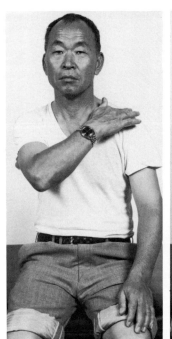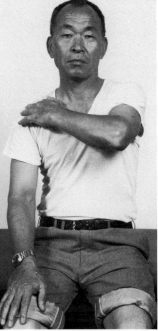

**Fig. 2.7** *Excessive left-sided shoulder girdle elevation in frame 2 indicates a poorly controlled relationship between shoulder girdle elevators and shoulder flexors. He is compensating for poor control of deltoid. Frame 1 demonstrates normal function of his intact R. arm.*

### Hand

- Difficulty grasping with wrist in extension and radial deviation.

- Difficulty extending the metacarpo-phalangeal joints with the interphalangeal joints in some flexion in order to position the fingers for grasping and releasing an object.

- Difficulty with abduction and rotation of the thumb for grasp and release.

- Inability to release an object without flexing the wrist (Fig. 2.8).

- Excessive extension of fingers and thumb on release (usually with some wrist flexion).

- Tendency to pronate the forearm excessively while holding on to or picking up an object (i.e. whenever fingers flex).

- Inability to hold different objects while moving the arm.

- Excessive ulnar deviation while using the hand.

- Difficulty cupping the hand (Fig. 2.9).

In addition, there are five common sequelae of stroke, all of which are probably preventable.

- Habitual posturing of the limb.
- Neglect of the affected arm.
- Compensation with the intact arm.
- Use of the intact arm to move the affected arm.
- Contracture of the soft tissues of the shoulder and/or wrist.

Fig. 2.8

Fig. 2.9

**Fig. 2.8** *This man lacks control of his wrist and finger extensors. His attempts to release the bottle are accompanied by wrist flexion.* **Fig. 2.9** *Notice the abnormal posture of the thumb and the flatness of the ulnar side of the hand.*

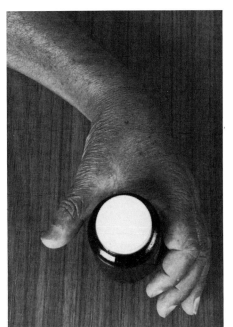

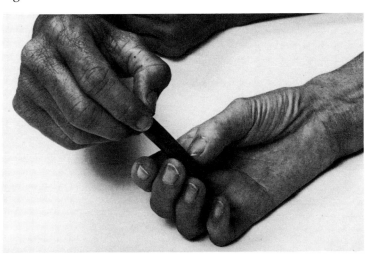

## Analysis of the Painful Shoulder

It must be understood that, as a result of depressed motor activity around the shoulder, the surrounding musculature, which normally controls and protects the anatomical relationship of the gleno-humeral joint, is inactive. The gleno-humeral joint is not a stable joint, even when the muscles controlling it are functional; when they are inactive, its instability is total.

Soft tissue injury with resultant pain, stiffness and subluxation will usually result from three mechanical factors: (a) pinching of soft tissue against the acromion, (b) friction of soft tissue against bone, and (c) traction to soft tissue. These mechanical factors are brought about by the following: passive range of motion exercises; exercises which tend to force abduction without external rotation; exercises which involve movement from a position of internal rotation and flexion, into elevation and abduction, then into external rotation and extension; the effect of gravity plus the weight of the flaccid arm; pulling on the limb to position the patient; rolling on to the paretic shoulder.

In addition to these factors, there is very often a failure to use the appropriate means of eliciting muscular activity and of training motor control around the shoulder. The pathological conditions which develop include degeneration of the acromio-clavicular joint, bicipital tendinitis, bursitis, coracoiditis, and supraspinatus tendinitis,[2] Several authors[2,3] describe the occurrence of brachial plexus lesion following stroke, caused by traction on the unprotected shoulder and resulting in true muscle paralysis which may take 8 to 12 months or more to recover, if it recovers at all.

The mechanism of the painful shoulder is discussed in some detail by Najenson and his colleagues,[4] Cailliet,[2] and Griffin and Reddin.[5]

One of the major causes of a painful, stiff shoulder is the use of **passive exercises.** Passive range of motion exercises, because they cannot be controlled by the inactive muscles surrounding the joint, will allow or force an abnormal relationship between humerus and scapula because they involve movement at the gleno-humeral joint without the corresponding and necessary movement of the shoulder girdle. They will therefore damage the soft tissues around the gleno-humeral joint. In addition, many stroke patients are elderly, and with increasing age degenerative changes develop within the rotator cuff[6] and predispose the shoulder to injury through passive movement.

Passive range of motion exercises include not only movements done by therapists or nurses, but also pulley exercises and passive ranging done by the patient himself using his intact arm. These exercises are usually done with the objective of preventing stiffness and soft tissue contracture. However, the patient will not develop a stiff shoulder if damage to the soft tissues is avoided and if, early following stroke, the therapist stimulates muscle activity with the arm in elevation (see Fig. 2.11).

Any complaint of pain from a patient should be analysed to establish a cause so that the necessary therapy can be commenced. Unfortunately, the therapist may react to pain and stiffness in the hemiplegic patient by stepping up passive movements in the belief that inactivity is causing the pain. This causes further trauma and increases the symptoms. These problems of musculo-skeletal origin should be diagnosed and analysed, and the therapy which would normally be given to a patient with such problems should be instituted as soon as possible. For example, if **pain** is the problem, treatment may include peripheral joint mobilisation,[7] interferential or transcutaneous nerve stimulation (T.N.S.). If **chronic inflammation** exists, heat or ultrasound may stimulate a more normal repair process. There are two possible components of **joint stiffness**: (i) adaptive tissue contracture secondary to disuse, and (ii) adhesions between normally free-sliding structures. The former will improve if the patient practises the movement outlined in this Programme, within a gradually increasing pain-free range. The latter will respond to peripheral joint mobilisation in addition to the practice of appropriate movements.

### STEPS 2 AND 3    PRACTICE OF UPPER LIMB FUNCTION

In general, the literature suggests that rehabilitation of upper limb function is unsuccessful, a large proportion of patients never re-establishing effective use of the arm and many of them developing a painful shoulder[2-4,8-16] for a variety of different reasons. It is probable that this is an unnecessary state of affairs and is largely due to inappropriate treatment techniques and a tendency to 'wait' for obvious signs of recovery before giving any active therapy.[14]

Leverage and the pull of gravity are two important factors to consider in the stimulation of upper limb function. Motor activity can be elicited early with the patient in supine with his arm in elevation (see Fig. 2.11). Frequently, muscles first contract eccentrically rather than concentrically, and in a particular part of their range, usually within the inner half of range. The therapist should not attempt to elicit motor activity around the shoulder with the patient's arm by his side, either in sitting or lying, as the muscles required to lift the limb are at a mechanical disadvantage.

Another important factor to consider is the way in which muscles normally function. Individual muscles or parts of muscles function with other muscles in an almost infinite variety of combinations, depending upon the activity being performed. Therefore, following stroke, a muscle may be encouraged to contract as part of one particular motor programme before it will contract as part of another. If a muscle cannot contract for its prime mover function, it may be able to contract as a synergist or fixator.

The first part of this section is relevant for the patient who, early after his stroke, apparently has little or no motor activity in the upper limb. The objective is to discover what motor activity exists by giving particular muscles the opportunity to contract as they normally would for a particular function, to point out to the patient what he can do and to encourage and to help him to extend his abilities. The therapist and nurse do not need to do passive range of motion exercises to maintain joint range, as the activities outlined below will not allow soft tissue contracture or joint stiffness to occur.

The following points should be kept in mind throughout this part of the Programme.

- Arm movements, including movements of the hand, must be stimulated early following stroke. Hand movements must not be left until there is some recovery of function around the shoulder, as suggested by some authors.[17] Recovery does **not** take place from proximal to distal, as is sometimes suggested, nor is it necessary to have control of the shoulder before attempting to regain control of the hand.

- Upper limb function is made up of very complex combinations of muscle action and every combination is used in normal everyday activities. As soon as isolated muscle action is elicited, this must be practised and extended into meaningful actions, with the patient gaining control over increasing ranges of a movement, changing to other movements which also require the muscle to contract in its prime mover, synergist and fixator roles, shifting from concentric to eccentric in different parts of range and at various speeds.

- All muscle activity unnecessary to the movement being attempted must be eliminated consciously by the patient. This includes movements of the intact side of the body (including the 'fidgeting' seen in some patients) and muscular activity in the affected arm which is not necessary for the particular movement or activity being practised. Elimination of unnecessary muscle activity allows the development of motor control and, in the case of unnecessary activity of the affected arm, appears to minimise the development of the flexor overactivity seen in some patients.

- Gross patterns of movements of the upper limb should be avoided as these will not allow either the therapist or the patient to be aware of any minimal muscle activity present and they will tend to encourage only the more active muscles (that is, those which tend to become overactive) to contract, and they may cause trauma around the shoulder (for example, bicipital tendinitis).[2]

- Activity should be elicited at first in the position of greatest advantage to the muscle. For example, in supine, arm flexed at 90° for the deltoid muscle.

- It is important that the therapist does not support the limb once sufficient muscle activity has been retrained. The support required when there is insufficient muscle activity is changed to guidance as soon as possible.

- If a muscle does not contract in a particular set of conditions, vary the conditions. For example, change the speed of movement, the relationship to gravity, etc.

- Muscles must not be allowed to contract incorrectly. That is, exercises should not be given which stimulate muscles to contract concentrically throughout an entire range of movement when this is unnatural in terms of the limb's changing relationship to gravity. An example of the latter is the change in muscle activity involved when the arm is moved from the side to above the head in the supine position.

● The patient should not be allowed or encouraged to practise movements which are part of an abnormal synergy and which have no functional significance. For example, he must not be given a rubber ball to squeeze as this encourages habituation of flexor activity, is usually combined with wrist flexion and pronation and therefore aids the development of a fixed flexion posture.

● Should flexor overactivity interfere with the training of arm movements and this cannot be overcome by conscious control, the cycle of overactivity and misplaced effort will need to be overcome by other means. Figure 2.10 illustrates a movement (see footnote on p. 33) which stimulates more appropriate motor activity and therefore decreases excessive flexor activity.

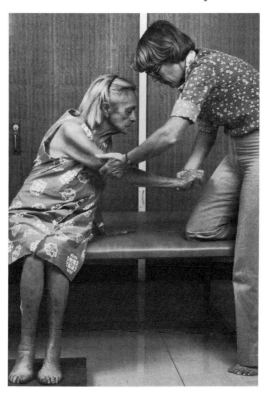

**Fig. 2.10** *The patient practises reaching sideways to touch the therapist's leg or the plinth. Emphasis should be on reaching out with the heel of the hand as this goal elicits wrist extensor activity. Therapist must ensure that the shoulder is not being depressed.*

● The therapist should not think in terms of strengthening muscles. The objective is to stimulate muscle activity and to train the patient to control this activity for function. As he practises controlled limb use, he will acquire the appropriate muscular strength and endurance relatively easily.

● Bilateral movements should be avoided until the patient regains control over the affected limb. Bilateral movements appear to reinforce movements of the intact limb at the expense of the affected limb and, if they are non-mirror actions, they probably cause a high degree of inter-hemispheric interference.[18] Diller[19] has observed that bilateral movements deteriorate the performance of both the intact and the affected hand. He cites studies which support his observation that this deterioration in performance is seen after both active and passive movements.

- Doing a movement passively for the patient should be avoided. Although it is useful to perform a particular movement passively in order to help the patient to understand what is required of him, persistence with this passive demonstration probably prevents him from eliciting any muscular activity by interfering with his attempts. It makes it impossible for the therapist to recognise any muscle activity which may occur and to feed back to the patient this information which is essential to the learning process. Furthermore, passive movements probably play little part in promoting motor learning. The information derived from passive movement is different from that derived from active movement.

### To Elicit Muscular Activity and Train Motor Control around the Shoulder

*Supine, therapist lifts the patient's arm and supports it in forward flexion. Patient attempts to reach up towards ceiling (Fig. 2.11).*

NOTE
This is to encourage shoulder girdle protraction and may also be done in side lying.

INSTRUCTIONS
'Reach up towards the ceiling.'
'Think about using your shoulder.'
'Now let your shoulder go back on to the bed.'

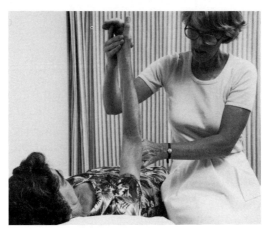

**Fig. 2.11** *This woman is practising reaching upwards. The therapist is holding the arm in the correct alignment.*

CHECK

Ensure scapula rotates—it may have to be moved passively into position during the first few attempts.

Do not allow forearm to pronate or gleno-humeral joint to internally rotate and do not hold the arm in these positions.

Do not allow the patient to retract the shoulder actively—the return movement should be eccentric.

*Supine, therapist lifts patient's arm and supports it in foward flexion. She stimulates muscular activity by asking patient to attempt parts of various activities, for example: (i) to take his hand to his head (Fig. 2.12); (ii) to take his hand above his head to the pillow (Fig. 2.13). This is an exploratory procedure, both therapist and patient trying to elicit muscular activity in certain key muscles (Fig. 2.14), particularly in deltoid and triceps brachii.*

NOTE

While only minimal muscular activity is present around the shoulder, the patient may complain of pain in the shoulder when the arm is raised to 90°. This may be due to nipping of soft tissues between the humeral head and acromion. It is usually relieved if the therapist separates the joint surfaces **minimally**. This is discontinued as soon as it is no longer necessary.

(i) INSTRUCTIONS

'See if you can take your hand down to your forehead—gently—don't let your hand drop. Now lift it up a little.'

CHECK

Do not allow patient to pronate forearm.

Assist patient to control position joint.

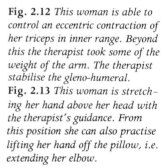

**Fig. 2.12** *This woman is able to control an eccentric contraction of her triceps in inner range. Beyond this the therapist took some of the weight of the arm. The therapist stabilise the gleno-humeral.*

**Fig. 2.13** *This woman is stretching her hand above her head with the therapist's guidance. From this position she can also practise lifting her hand off the pillow, i.e. extending her elbow.*

Fig. 2.12                    Fig. 2.13

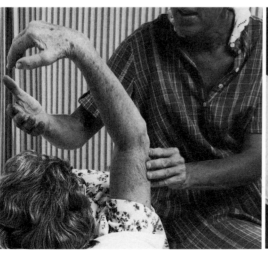

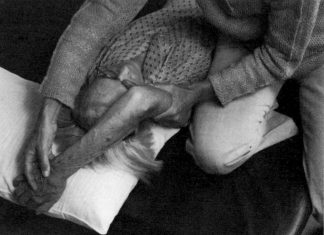

(ii) INSTRUCTIONS

'See if you can take your hand above your head to the pillow. I'll help you. Now try to stretch your arm above your head.'

CHECK

Do not allow patient to pronate forearm.

Do not allow shoulder to abduct.

Check that scapula movement is correct.

(a)

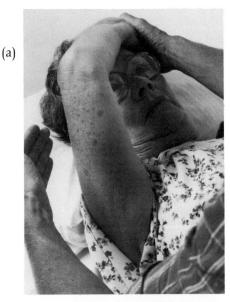

**Fig. 2.14(a)** *The therapist holds this woman's hand on her head while she practises controlling an eccentric contraction of the shoulder flexors,* **(b)** *In this photograph, she has gone on to lift her arm and move her hand to her head, then move her arm back to the therapist's leg,* **(c)** *She has difficulty controlling supination and needs to practise supination separately. This practice is followed by taking her hand to her head again.*

(b)

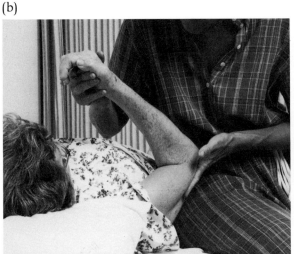

(c)

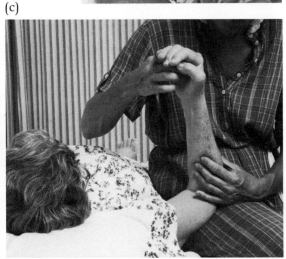

As soon as the patient has some control over such muscles as deltoid, pectorals and triceps, he should progress to the following activities.

*Patient practises holding his arm in forward flexion and moving it within an ever-increasing range, always maintaining control (Fig. 2.15).*

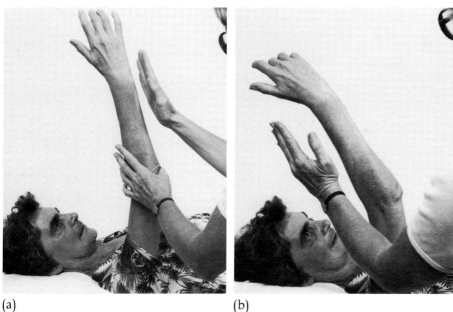

(a)                                        (b)

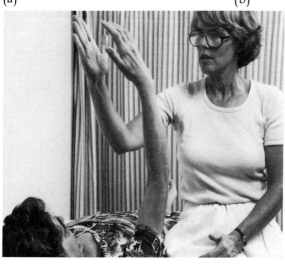

(c)

**Fig. 2.15** *This woman is improving control over flexion and extension of the arm. In* (a) *she needs some assistance to keep her arm from abducting. In* (b) *she needs only guidance as she follows the directional cue given by the therapist. Part of her practice involves switching from a concentric contraction of her shoulder flexor muscles to an eccentric contraction of her extensors as the movement changes direction. In* (c) *she shows how she can now control abduction and adduction of her arm in forward flexion.*

INSTRUCTIONS
'Stretch up with your hand—keep your elbow straight.'
'See if you can follow my hand.'

CHECK
Do not allow forearm to pronate, elbow to flex, or shoulder to internally rotate excessively.

Followed by:

*Sitting at a table, patient practises lowering his arm and lifting it up again (Fig. 2.16). He should work within the range he can control, gradually increasing it. When he can control his shoulder above 90°, he practises raising and lowering his arm below 90° in small but increasing ranges of movement, until he can move his arm from his side, both in flexion and in abduction, and in sitting as well as in standing.*

INSTRUCTIONS
'Take your arm down to the pillow. Don't let it drop.'
'Now reach up to touch my hand.'

CHECK
Do not allow elevation of the shoulder girdle as a substitute for abduction or flexion of the shoulder.
Do not allow elbow to flex.

**Fig. 2.16** *This woman is practising controlling an eccentric contraction of her shoulder flexors. She needs to be reminded to keep her shoulders level and her head straight.*

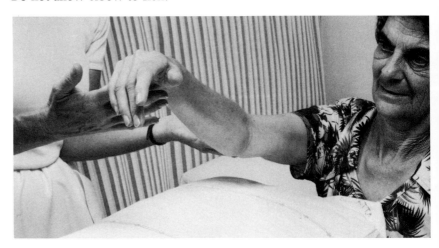

## To Maintain Length of Wrist and Finger Flexors

*With the patient in sitting or standing, therapist helps him to keep his hands on the wall, with his arm abducted/flexed forward at 90°. Therapist helps him place his arm in this position. Some horizontal pressure through his arm will make him more aware of its position and prevent his hand from sliding down the wall. Initially, the therapist will need to hold the elbow extended. In this position, the patient practises bending and straightening his elbow in order to improve control over his elbow extensors and, as he regains some shoulder and elbow control, he practises turning his trunk and head (Fig. 2.17).*

NOTE
It is important to prevent contracture of wrist and finger flexors as this will cause pain and interfere with training of hand function. In the early stages following stroke, this activity also helps to prevent neglect of the

upper limb by increasing the patient's visual and spatial awareness of the limb. It is also used to train muscle control around the shoulder and elbow.

INSTRUCTIONS
'Let your elbow bend a little. Straighten your elbow by pushing the heel of your hand into the wall gently.'
Progress to:
'Keep your hand on the wall and turn your body to face the front/side. Make sure your hand doesn't slip.'

CHECK
Do not allow hand to slide down wall.
Make sure thumb is extended
Draw his attention to his hand. Make sure weight is on both feet and shoulders are level.
Correct standing or sitting alignment.

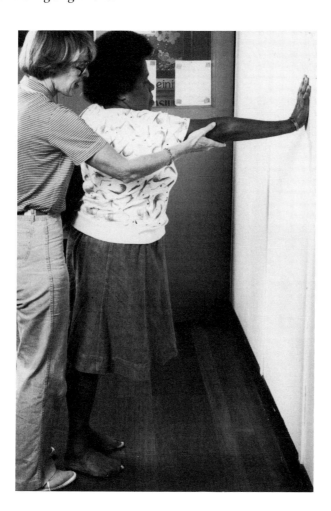

**Fig. 2.17** *The therapist helps this woman to keep her hand on the wall while asking her to turn her trunk and head to the left.*

### To Elicit Muscular Activity and Train Motor Control of the Hand

### To Stimulate Wrist Extension and Radial Deviation

*Patient sitting with arm supported on the table, forearm in mid position, fingers and thumb around cylindrical object. He attempts to extend wrist while holding it in some radial deviation (Fig. 2.18).*

NOTE
Patient will be more successful at extending his wrist if he first practises radial deviation (Fig. 2.18a).

INSTRUCTIONS
'Try to lift the glass off the table.'
Progress to:
'Take your hand back.'

CHECK
Do not allow elbow to flex.
Correct tendency for wrist to flex when it should be extending.

**Fig. 2.18(a)** *This woman is practising radial deviation of her wrist. Therapist assists by keeping her wrist in extension.* **(b)** *This man is practising extending his wrist while holding it in some radial deviation. The therapist helps him to keep his fingers around the jar.*

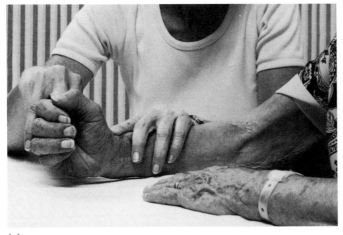

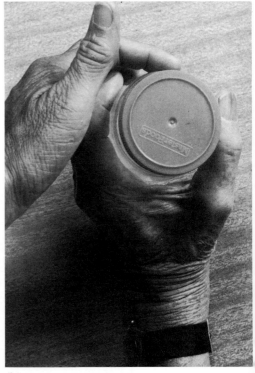

(a)

(b)

*As above with forearm in pronation and a cylindrical object in the hand.*

INSTRUCTION
'Lift your hand off the table.'

CHECK
Do not allow elbow to flex.
Correct tendency for wrist to ulnar deviate.
Patient must not extend wrist with fingers extended—therapist may need to assist him to hold the object.
Attention should be directed to wrist movement. The patient should be stopped from grasping too firmly as this may prevent him from extending the wrist.

NOTE
Patient should also practise, with forearm in both positions, lifting object, moving it backwards and forwards, or from one side to the other. Attention to this goal may be more successful in eliciting wrist movement than attempts merely to lift the object up.

## To Stimulate Supination

*Fingers around cylindrical object, patient attempts to supinate forearm.*

INSTRUCTIONS
'Try to turn your palm to face upwards—don't worry about holding the object—I'll help you.'

CHECK
Do not allow forearm to lift off table.
Correct tendency for wrist to flex and ulnar deviate.

## To Stimulate Palmar Abduction and Rotation of the Thumb (Opposition)

*Therapist holds forearm in mid position and wrist in extension, while patient attempts to grasp and release a cylindrical object (Fig. 2.19). The therapist will need to guide the movement until there is some muscular control (Fig. 2.19a).*

NOTE
The therapist guides the patient's hand towards the object. This action, with its intention to take hold of the object, may stimulate the thumb to abduct and the fingers to extend at the metacarpo-phalangeal joints.

INSTRUCTIONS
'Try to open your hand to take this. I'll help you.'
'Now, let it go.'

CHECK
Do not allow wrist to flex or forearm to pronate.
Wrist should be kept in some radial deviation.
When he has some thumb movement, make sure he abducts the thumb during release and does not slide it up the object (Fig. 2.19b).
Make sure the thumb posture is correct, that is, pad of thumb grasps object, not medial border (Fig. 2.19c).

**Fig. 2.19(a)** *Therapist holds thumb, fingers and wrist in a posture which enables the patient to grasp the object.* **(b)** *This woman, in releasing the bandage, has extended her thumb laterally instead of abducting it. She needs to practise the component of palmar abduction.* **(c)** *It is important that in all hand activities the therapist ensures the correct posture of the thumb and fingers. Here, during practice of wrist movement, the patient is holding his thumb incorrectly. It is flexed at the metacarpal joint instead of being abducted in a palmar direction.*

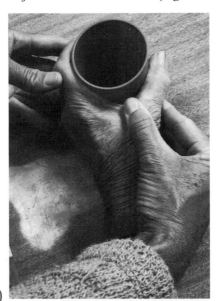

(a)

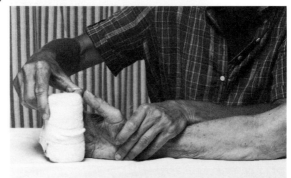

(b)

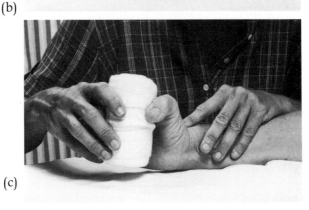

(c)

## To Stimulate Opposition of Radial and Ulnar Sides of Hand (Cupping of the Hand)

*Forearm in supination, patient practises opposing thumb and other fingers, particularly fourth and fifth fingers (Fig. 2.20). Therapist demonstrates how the palm of the hand should cup.*

INSTRUCTIONS
'Touch the tip of your little finger to your thumb. Make sure you move your finger as well as your thumb.'
'Cup your hand.'

CHECK
Make sure movement occurs at carpo-metacarpal joint and not just at metacarpo-phalangeal joint.
Tips of fingers and thumb should touch.

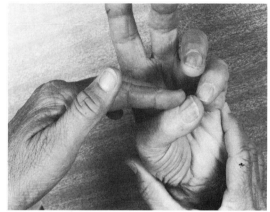

**Fig. 2.20** *Practice of opposition between thumb and little finger. Therapist guides the cupping movement.*

## To Train Control over Manipulation of Objects

Below are some suggestions indicating some of the varied activities the patient should practise.

*Patient practises picking up various small objects between thumb and each finger (Fig. 2.21). He can go on to picking these out of a bowl and releasing them into another bowl, supinating his hand while holding the object, etc.*

**Fig. 2.21** *Therapist needs to assist this patient to control the correct posture of the hand.*

INSTRUCTIONS
'Pick this up and put it here.'

CHECK
Make sure patient uses the pad of the thumb for holding object, not the medial side.
Make sure the wrist is not actively flexing while releasing the object (see Fig. 2.8), although depending on arm position, the wrist may need to be held in a flexed position.

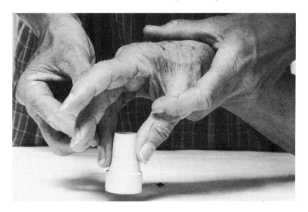

*Patient practises picking up polystyrene cup around the rim without deforming it (Fig. 2.22). He should practise picking it up, holding it while moving his arm, and releasing it. He should do this with his hand close to his body, away from his body, and in conjunction with the other hand (for example, pouring water from one cup to another).*

**NOTE**
This will train dynamaesthesia.

**INSTRUCTIONS**
'Pick up this cup—don't change its shape.'

**CHECK**
Do not allow patient to grip inappropriately, that is, so firmly that he deforms it or so gently that he drops it.

**Fig. 2.22** *This man is concentrating on controlling his grasp so as not to deform the cup. He should also practise holding the cup at its side. He should be reminded to keep his shoulders level.*

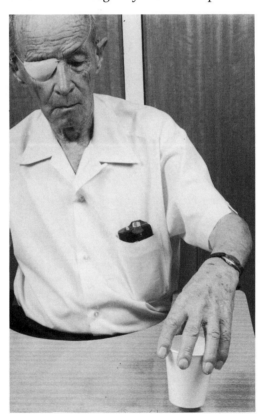

*With forearm in mid position, patient practises lifting cylindrical object up, extending wrist, putting it down, lifting it up again, flexing wrist, putting it down.*

**CHECK**
Do not allow patient to let object go—he should hold on throughout.
Do not allow forearm to pronate.

*Patient practises picking a piece of paper from his opposite shoulder (Fig. 2.23).*

CHECK
Do not allow forearm to pronate.

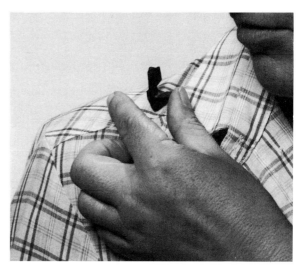

**Fig. 2.23** *Practice of picking an object off the shoulder.*

In order to use the hand effectively, it is necessary to have a fine degree of control over the shoulder. The following are some examples of how to increase complexity.

- Reaching forward to pick up or touch an object.
- Reaching sideways to pick up an object from a table and transferring it to a table in front.
- Grasping and releasing an object with the arm stretched out behind (see Fig. 5.15).
- Using two hands together to manipulate objects.

CHECK
Correct any tendency to use the incorrect musculature or an inappropriate degree of motor activity, for example excessive elevation of the shoulder girdle as a substitute for forward flexion or abduction of the shoulder.

The patient should never practise what he can already do. If he finds a particular component of a movement difficult or if the therapist sees he is performing a particular component in an abnormal manner, he should practise this with guidance in as many ways and for as many different activities as possible.

When training the affected limb to perform a function which is normally bimanual (for example, in the use of tools such as knife and fork), the patient may use his affected hand more efficiently if he also uses the intact hand for the relevant part of the task. This must be done without overflow of activity into inappropriate muscle groups and is particularly effective for the person who is regaining motor control in his hand but who needs to practise more complex tasks.

For the patient to learn to manipulate a particular tool (toothbrush, comb, tools of trade) requires from the therapist a specific analysis of each function to determine the missing components. This means that the therapist should know which are the essential components for the use of that tool. An example of how to train a patient in the use of cutlery is given below.

## To Improve the Use of Cutlery

Throughout practice, the therapist must constantly compare the patient's performance with the normal (Fig. 2.24). Manipulative activities are very complex, yet a patient will often be able to improve his performance quickly if the therapist can pick out the major factor interfering with that performance. Certain problems are particularly common and require specific training.

**Fig. 2.24(a)** *and* **(c)** *illustrate the method of holding cutlery which is being trained below,* **(b)** *shows the position of the knife and fork in the palm of the hand.*

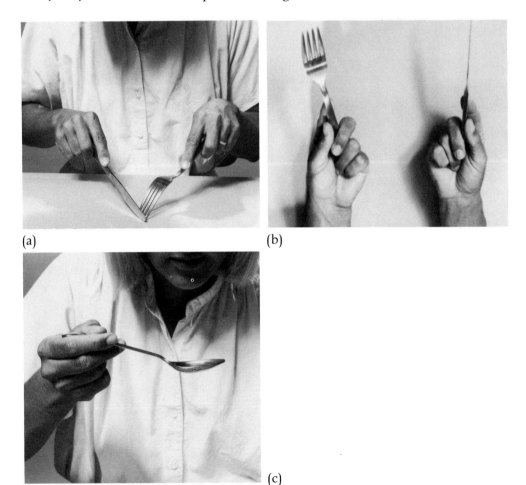

(a)

(b)

(c)

**The Fork**

1. Difficulty moving fork into position in hand once it is picked up.

*With forearm in pronation, patient practises turning small objects over in the palm of his hand using his fingers and thumb.*

Followed by:

*Patient practises picking up fork and moving it into position in his hand.*

2. Difficulty holding fork between thumb, index and middle fingers (Fig. 2.24a).

*Patient practises picking up small objects between thumb, index and middle fingers.*

Followed by:

*Patient uses fork with therapist's guidance.*

CHECK
Do not allow him to pronate forearm excessively.

3. Difficulty holding fork between ring and little fingers and palm (Fig. 2.24b).

*Patient practises picking up a jelly bean between thumb and ring finger, thumb and little finger, supinating and pronating the forearm while holding the object, putting it in a bowl.*

CHECK
Make sure he picks up with tips of thumb and fingers. Followed by:

*Patient uses fork with therapist's guidance.*

CHECK
Do not allow him to pronate forearm excessively.

4. Difficulty holding fork while pressing down on food.

*Patient practises using fork to hold food and to pick it up with therapist's guidance.*

CHECK
Do not allow patient to pronate forearm excessively.
Make sure he can make the change from active flexion while pressing down on fork to active extension as he lifts food from the plate or moves fork elsewhere on plate.

NOTE
Whenever the patient practises manipulating his fork, he will do better if he holds a knife in his other hand, and if he has before him a plate with food (for example, cheese) on it.

### The Knife

The difficulties listed above are also seen when using a knife and should be trained in a similar manner. Below are some examples of difficulties specifically related to the use of a knife.

1. Difficulty holding knife while cutting meat.

*Patient practises using knife to cut food with therapist's guidance.*

CHECK
Do not allow him to press down too hard.
Do not allow him to pronate forearm excessively.

2. Difficulty pushing food towards fork.

*Patient practises using knife to push food towards fork.*

CHECK
Do not allow him to pronate excessively.

### The Spoon

1. Difficulty moving spoon into position in hand once it is picked up.

*With forearm in supination, patient practises touching thumb and each fingertip separately as quickly as possible while maintaining accuracy.*

*With forearm in supination, patient practises turning over a small object in his hand.*

2. Difficulty adjusting grasp in order to keep bowl of spoon level as it is raised from plate to mouth (Fig. 2.24c).

*Patient practises moving his arm while holding spoon. Spoon should contain fluid, as this will be a useful monitoring device for him.*

Followed by:

*Patient practises taking spoon (with fluid) to mouth.*

CHECK
Do not allow him to take his head down to the spoon.

**STEP 4**       TRANSFERENCE OF LEARNING INTO DAILY LIFE

If the patient is to recover upper limb function, there are three points which must be considered.

1. He must not suffer **secondary soft tissue injury**. It is possible for the shoulder to be injured by any member of the staff, by a relative and by the patient himself. Nurses, therapists, porters and doctors must not pull on the patient's arm to move him about. Passive movements to check for joint range limitation or with the objective of maintaining or increasing joint range will damage the soft tissues around the paretic shoulder joint. The patient should not be allowed to move his affected arm passively and he should not be given pulley exercises. Both activities fail to take into account normal scapulo-humeral rhythm and therefore increase the likelihood of soft tissue injury in the shoulder region.

2. He must not be allowed or encouraged to develop 'learned non-use'[20] of his affected arm, by performing activities which involve movement of the affected limb by the intact limb or by moving about using only the intact limbs. During these activities, the patient will be attending only to the arm which can move and not at all to the affected one. Several studies with de-afferentated and brain-damaged monkeys[20,21] indicate that unrestrained use of the intact limb may be a major factor in failure to recover function in the affected limb. If the animal's intact limb is restrained and he is trained to use the affected limb, he regains effective use of this limb. The possibility of physically restraining the affected limb of a human for short periods of the day has recently been investigated in one patient[22] but, as the authors point out, further research is needed. However, therapist, nurse and relatives should discourage, using verbal and cognitive restraint, any unnecessary and compensatory activity in the intact limb. The patient should understand the reason for this restraint and should try not to use his intact arm unnecessarily.

3. The patient must not be given a ball to squeeze as this will encourage overactivity in the flexor muscles.

During the day the patient should practise particular components or movements on which the therapist considers he should concentrate. Movements which are too difficult to practise on his own can be practised mentally (see p. 166). However, the therapist should, whenever possible, teach a relative or friend how to help the patient practise movements or movement components.

Until the patient has regained antigravity control of the muscles around the shoulder, his arm, when he is sitting, should be supported so the head of the humerus is held in the glenoid cavity. This can be accomplished if the patient has his arm supported on pillows with his elbow close to his side. He should be encouraged to sit symmetrically with shoulders level, as depression of the shoulder girdle alters the angle of the glenoid cavity and predisposes the shoulder joint to subluxation (Fig. 2.25). He should sometimes sit with arms supported on a table in front of him as this is a natural position, gives him an alternative to sitting with his arm by his side, and gives him the opportunity to practise mentally and physically the manipulative activities he has been practising with the therapist.

The use of different types of **sling** is questionable. [23-28] Certainly, they can be remarkably ineffectual. The authors examined radiologically the effects of five different types of sling on a particular patient with subluxation of the shoulder. None of the slings made any difference at all. Figure 2.25 illustrates the effect of one of these slings. There appears to be no sling which has been shown by radiographic study to be effective. However, a new harness has recently been devised* and is being investigated for effectiveness. It is important that a method is found which protects the paretic shoulder from injury and traction while the patient walks around. There must be a balance between protecting the shoulder from injury, preventing neglect or 'learned non-use' of the limb, and ensuring the best position for the regaining of motor control. The major objective remains the early recovery of motor control around an undamaged shoulder.

The value of hand splints following stroke is a controversial point and Einbond[29] and Neuhaus and colleagues[30] describe the inconsistent and confusing rationale expressed by both the non-splinting group of therapists and the splinting group. This confusion is probably an illustration of the lack of understanding both of the problems of upper limb function following stroke and of the proper objectives of rehabilitation. Furthermore, the pathophysiology of stroke seems to be assumed to be the same as for brain damage following head injury and for

**Fig. 2.25** *Note the difference in the position of the head of the humerus in these two pictures. Radiography of five different slings showed no effect upon the degree of subluxation,* **(a)** *illustrates one of these slings,* **(b)** *illustrates the effect of supporting the same patient's arm on pillows.*

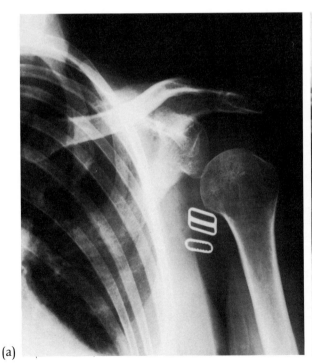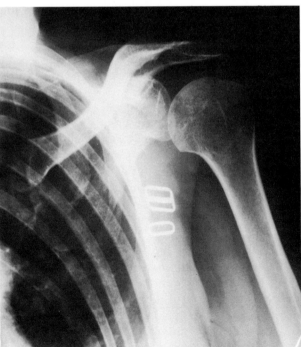

(a)

*Hook hemi-harness. Created by the Orthopaedic Equipment Company, Bourbon, Indiana, USA 46504, in conjunction with the August E. Hook Physical Rehabilitation Center.

cerebral palsy. Hence, the motor problems and their treatment are assumed, incorrectly, to be the same.

Unfortunately, much splinting is applied by therapists who have negative expectations of recovery of upper limb function. Hence, such splinting may actually prevent the patient regaining any motor control by preventing use of the hand.

Splinting, if it needs to be considered, must fulfil the objective of enabling muscles to regain function, by putting joints in a position which favours the relearning of certain movement components. If, for example, moulded plastic is used to hold the thumb in a position of some palmar abduction in the early stages before the person has regained control of the thumb, and if this splint is small enough not to interfere with the person's practice of hand movement, then it may well be effective in helping the person to regain control of thumb abduction, grasp and release.

## REFERENCES

1. Roland P. E. (1973). Lack of appreciation of compressibility adynamaesthesia and akinaesthesia. *J. neurol. Sci*; **20**:51–61.
2. Cailliet R. (1980). *The Shoulder in Hemiplegia*. Philadelphia: F. A. Davis.
3. Kaplan P. E., Meredith J., Taft G. and Betts H. B. (1977). Stroke and brachial plexus injury: a difficult problem. *Arch. phys. Med*; **58**, 9:415–18.
4. Najenson T., Yacubovich E. and Pikielni S. (1971). Rotator cuff injury in shoulder joints of hemiplegic patients. *Scand. J. Rehab. Med*; **3**:131–7.
5. Griffin J. and Reddin G. (1981). Shoulder pain in patients with hemiplegia. *Phys. Therapy* **61**, 7:1041–5.
6. Mosley H. F. (1963). The vascular supply of the rotator cuff. *Surg. Clin. N. Amer*; **43**:1521–2.
7. Maitland G. D. (1977). *Peripheral Manipulation*, 2nd edn. London: Butterworths.
8. Caldwell C. B., Wilson D. J. and Braun R. M. (1969). Evaluation and treatment of the upper extremity in the hemiplegic stroke patient. *Clinical Orthopaedics and Related Research*; **63**:69–93.
9. Moskowitz H., Goodman C. R. and Smith E. (1969). Hemiplegic shoulder. *N.Y. St. J. Med*; **69**:548–50.
10. Loombs J. (1973). Facilitation techniques in hemiplegia: treatment of the arm. *Physiotherapy Canada*; **25**, 5:283–8.
11. Mossman P. L. (1976). *A Problem-Orientated Approach to Stroke Rehabilitation*. Illinois: Charles C. Thomas.
12. Davis S. W., Petrillo C. R., Rodolfo D. E. and Chu D. S. (1977). Shoulder–hand syndrome in a hemiplegic population: a 5-year retrospective study. *Arch. phys. Med*; **58**: 353–6.
13. Brocklehurst J., Andrews K., Richards B. and Laycock P. J. (1978). How much physical therapy for patients with stroke? *Brit. med J*; 20 May:1307–10.
14. Johnstone M. (1978). *Restoration of Motor Function in the Stroke Patient*. London: Churchill Livingstone.
15. Jensen E. M. (1980). The hemiplegic shoulder. *Scand. J. Rehab. Med*, Suppl; 7:113–119.
16. Carr J. and Shepherd R. (1982). The neglected upper limb following stroke. *Aust. J. Physiother*; in press.

17. Dardier E. (1980). *The Early Stroke Patient*. London: Baillière Tindall.
18. Stockmeyer S. (1981). Interference and Co-operation in Hemispheric Function. Paper given at *First Austral-Asian Physiotherapy Congress, Singapore*.
19. Diller L. (1970). Psychomotor and vocational rehabilitation. In *Behavioral Changes in Cerebrovascular Disease* (Benton A. L., ed.) pp. 81–116. New York: Harper and Row.
20. Taub E. (1980). Somato-sensory deafferentation research with monkeys: implications for rehabilitation medicine. In *Behavioral Psychology in Rehabilitation Medicine: Clinical Applications* (Ince L. P., ed.) pp. 371–401 Baltimore: Williams and Wilkins.
21. Yu J. (1976). Functional recovery with and without training following brain damage in experimental animals: a review. *Arch. phys. Med*; **57**:38–41.
22. Ostendorf C. G. and Wolf S. L. (1981). Effect of forced use of the upper extremity of a hemiplegic patient on changes in function. *Phys. Ther*; **61**:1022–28.
23. Voss D. (1969). Should patients with hemiplegia wear a sling? *Phys. Ther*; **49**:1030.
24. Braun R. M. (1969). Should patients with hemiplegia wear a sling? *Phys. Ther*; **49**:1029–30.
25. Hurd M. M., Farrell K. H. and Waylonis G. W. (1974). Shoulder sling for hemiplegia: friend or foe? *Arch. phys Med*; **55**:519–22.
26. Bobath B. (1978). *Adult Hemiplegia: Evaluation and Treatment*, 2nd edn. London: Heinemann Medical.
27. Wilson D. and Caldwell C. B. (1978). A treatment approach emphasizing upper extremity orthoses. *Phys. Ther*; **58**:313–20.
28. Neal M. R. and Williamson J. (1980). Collar sling for bilateral shoulder subluxation. *Amer. J. occup. Ther*; **34**:400–401.
29. Einbond A. (1978). *Survey of Occupational Therapists' Criteria for Splinting Hemiplegic Hands: Rational or Ritual?* Paper submitted in partial fulfillment of the requirement for the degree of Master of Science, available from Columbia University, New York.
30. Neuhaus B. E. *et al*. (1981). A survey of rationales for and against hand splinting in hemiplegia. *Amer. J. occup. Ther*; **35**:83–90.

# 3

# *Oro-facial function*

Oro-facial function comprises various activities, such as **swallowing, facial expression, ventilation** and **speech.** Following stroke, all these activities may be affected, interfering with eating, communication and socialisation. Oro-facial problems are embarrassing and frustrating and may affect relationships between the patient and his relatives and the staff. Remediation of these problems should therefore begin immediately, as they respond very quickly to early treatment.

In the first few days, it is the abnormal or ineffective **swallowing** which causes the greatest dysfunction. Drooling, aspiration and difficulty ingesting food result in a poor nutritional state and may lead to the provision of a nasogastric tube. It is particularly important that normal swallowing is retrained as soon as possible and that the use of a nasogastric tube is avoided. Nasogastric tube feeding is unpleasant and may cause hypersensitivity of the oral area. It leads to irritation of the mucous membrane, lack of stimulus to chew or move the tongue, and predisposes to oesophageal reflux.[1] As the patient is not taking food normally, he is deprived of the pleasurable stimuli of different types of food. More normal swallowing will occur once the patient has jaw and lip closure, a more mobile tongue and the stimulus of something to swallow.

### DESCRIPTION OF NORMAL SWALLOWING

Swallowing is a highly complex and integrated neuromuscular function.[2,3] The initial stage, the preparation of the bolus, is under voluntary control, but once the bolus is passed into the oral pharynx the second, or involuntary, stage of the act of swallowing begins. It is the contact of the bolus or saliva with the mucosa of the back of the tongue and pharynx which sets up the swallowing reflex. During the involuntary stage the food passes through the pharynx to the oesophagus, partly under the influence of gravity with the person in the erect position and partly due to the successive contraction of the constrictor muscles.

Food is taken into the mouth with the lips and is bitten by the front teeth. The tongue moves the food on to the molars and mixes the food with salivary secretions. The cheek, comprising the buccinator muscle, also assists in controlling the food in the mouth by pushing the food back on to the molars when the action of chewing tends to push it sideways.

The tongue selects the food that is sufficiently moistened for swallowing. The anterior part of the tongue is raised and pressed against the hard palate just behind the front teeth. The bolus is formed on the tongue and squeezed backwards towards the posterior oral cavity by movement of the tongue against the hard palate. This movement commences at the tip of the tongue and spreads back rapidly.[3] To help form the bolus, the soft palate closes down on to the back of the tongue. The bolus is passed into the oral pharynx through the palatoglossal arches by elevation of the posterior third of the tongue in a postero-superior direction. In swallowing fluids, the intrinsic muscles of the tongue are used to form a tunnel with the hard palate and to squirt fluid back through the mouth.

In preparation for swallowing, the hyoid bone is brought forward into a position of moderate elevation through the movements of the tongue. The lips and jaw are closed and the soft palate and uvula made tense to seal off the nasopharynx. The larynx is pulled upward behind the hyoid bone and towards the back of the tongue. This narrows the lumen of the larynx which helps to protect the respiratory tract. As the bolus reaches the epiglottis, some of it spills sideways descending on one or both sides of the larynx into the oesophagus. The pharynx is also pulled upwards over the bolus, propelling it a short distance into the oesophagus. Once the bolus enters the oesophagus it continues downward by peristaltic action. Breathing is inhibited momentarily during swallowing.

### ESSENTIAL COMPONENTS

- Jaw closure.
- Lip closure.
- Elevation of posterior third of tongue to close off posterior oral cavity.
- Elevation of lateral borders of tongue.

There are certain pre-requisites which are necessary for effective swallowing.

- Balanced sitting.
- Ability to move head independently of body.
- Normal threshold to sensation.
- Control of breathing in relation to swallowing.
- Normal reflex activity (the gag reflex is the only reflex normally present in the adult).

**STEP 1     ANALYSIS OF ORO-FACIAL FUNCTION**

Analysis of oro-facial function involves:

- observation of sitting position
- observation of movements of lips, jaw, cheeks
- intra-oral digital examination of tongue and cheeks (to test threshold to touch and to establish whether the tongue offers the normal resistance to movement)
- observation of eating and drinking.

## Difficulty with Swallowing

Lack of control over oro-facial musculature will result in:

- open jaw
- poor lip seal
- tongue too far forward and asymmetrically placed
- drooling
- immobile hypotonic tongue (tongue may look enlarged)
- food collecting between cheek and gums. Although this is often attributed to lack of muscular activity in the cheek (buccinator), a major factor is undoubtedly the immobility of the tongue.

Altered threshold to stimulation will result in:

- diminished awareness, which will cause difficulty keeping false teeth in place and a lack of awareness of saliva and food in the mouth, or
- hypersensitivity, which will be demonstrated by a hyperactive gag reflex, retraction of the tongue, and aversion to touch and to the presence of food in the mouth. This occurs as a secondary problem, due to fear of choking in untreated patients and after prolonged use of a nasogastric tube.

## Asymmetry of Facial Expression

This is the result of lack of motor control of the lower part of the face on the affected side, together with overactivity and unopposed activity of the face on the intact side. The upper third of the face receives bilateral innervation and therefore is not usually affected following stroke.

## Lack of Emotional Control

Although not an oro-facial problem *per se*, lack of control over the physical manifestations of the emotions is frequently seen in the early stages following stroke. This lack of control is demonstrated by outbursts of uncontrolled crying which are not necessarily related to sadness and which the patient has difficulty modifying or stopping. If the patient is not given a solution to this problem, it is very likely to persist and to interfere with his training programme, with his regaining of self-esteem and with his personal relationships.

### Poor Breathing Control

This may result from a combination of factors including poor control over the soft palate, or motor impersistence,[4,5] which is demonstrated by difficulty in taking a deep breath, holding the breath, and making a prolonged 'ah' sound on expiration.

### STEP 2    PRACTICE OF MISSING COMPONENTS

The most efficient position for swallowing, and therefore for eating, is sitting. The therapist should check the patient's sitting position and ensure that he is sitting with hips well back in the chair and with his head and trunk erect.

The patient who wears false teeth should be helped to put them in place. This will improve his appearance, reduce his embarrassment and prevent his gums from altering. His improved appearance will have a positive effect on the people around him.

The use of a spatula is not recommended in treatment because of its unpleasant texture and because the therapist's finger is a more effective tool for evaluating oral function.

The lips and intra-oral area are sensitive to temperature change. Ice, which is sometimes used to stimulate oral function, has in fact a numbing effect which increases the patient's difficulty in moving his tongue around his mouth or in knowing if his lips are closed or not. Sucking an ice block may also cause him to aspirate, as liquids are more easily aspirated than solids.[1]

In the techniques described below, most of which were devised by Mueller,[6] the therapist should not persist for too long with stimulation as the patient will tend to become desensitised and will fail to respond. For example, in training lip closure, the therapist should not use continuous or persistent stimulation but should use her finger briefly to indicate to the patient where he should concentrate his attention. Intra-oral techniques should be interrupted frequently, the fingers removed and the jaw held closed in order to allow the patient to swallow. Presence of saliva and closure of the jaw and lips will combine with the improved muscular activity of the tongue to trigger off swallowing.

## To Train Swallowing

### To Train Jaw Closure

*Tongue must be inside mouth. Therapist holds jaw closed with atlanto-occipital joint in the mid position (Fig. 3.1).*

NOTE
This technique should be performed throughout therapy sessions whenever necessary, that is, whenever jaw hangs open and whenever the patient needs to swallow.

INSTRUCTIONS
'Close your mouth.'
'Keep your teeth gently together.'

CHECK
Make sure not to push the atlanto-occipital joint into extension.

### To Train Lip Closure

*Therapist holds the jaw closed, using her finger to indicate to the patient the lip area which is not functioning (see Fig. 3.1).*

INSTRUCTIONS
'Keep your lips gently together.'

CHECK
Do not allow patient to suck on lower lip as this interferes with tongue movement for swallowing.
Do not encourage patient to pout.
Jaw must be closed.
Make sure nose is clear.

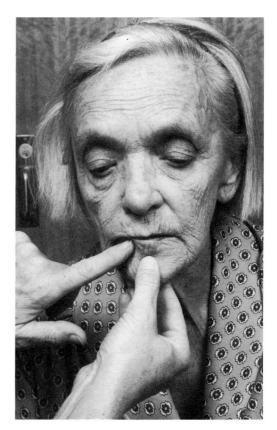

**Fig. 3.1** *Therapist holds the jaw closed and asks this woman to keep her lips gently together.*

### To Train Tongue Movement

*Therapist uses one or two fingers to give horizontal digital vibration to the anterior third of tongue with firm pressure downwards (Fig. 3.2). The amplitude of the vibratory movement should be small and the stimulation should last no longer than 5 seconds. The therapist withdraws her fingers and assists with jaw closure.*

INSTRUCTIONS
'Open your mouth. I'm going to stimulate your tongue to help you to swallow.'
'Now close your mouth.'

CHECK
Tell patient when he has swallowed—he may not know.
Make sure atlanto-occipital joint is not extended excessively.
Do not put fingers too far back on tongue.
Do not repeatedly ask the patient to swallow—swallowing in the absence of saliva requires effort.[7]

**Fig. 3.2** *Vibratory stimulation to the tongue in a horizontal direction with firm pressure downwards.*

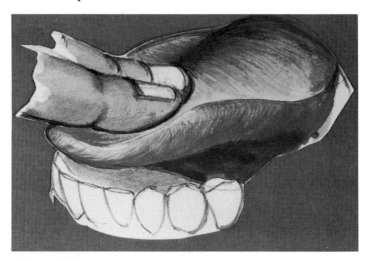

### To Elevate Posterior Third of Tongue

*Therapist uses index finger to give firm pressure to the anterior third of the tongue in a downwards direction to close off posterior oral cavity (Fig. 3.3). Follow immediately with lip and jaw closure as before.*

INSTRUCTIONS
'Open your mouth. I'm going to push down on your tongue to help you to swallow.'
'Now close your mouth.'
'Can you feel the back of your throat close off when you swallow?'

CHECK
As above.

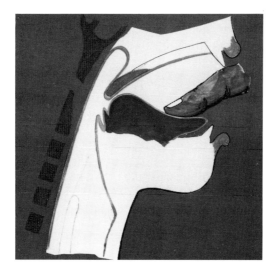

**Fig. 3.3** *Firm pressure downwards elicits elevation of the posterior third of the tongue to close off the posterior oral cavity.*

## To Elevate Lateral Margins of Tongue

*Therapist gives digital vibration inwards and upwards in a diagonal direction, with middle finger placed under the lateral margin of the tongue (Fig. 3.4). The amplitude of the vibratory movement should be small, and the stimulation should last no longer than 5 seconds. Follow immediately with lip and jaw closure as before.*

INSTRUCTIONS
'Open your mouth. I'm going to stimulate your tongue to help you to swallow.'
'Now close your mouth.'

CHECK
As above.
Finger must be under tongue and along side of velum.

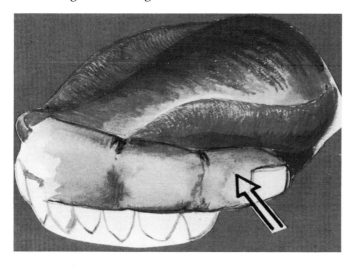

**Fig. 3.4** *Finger lies alongside the velum. Stimulation is given inwards towards the velum and upwards.*

## To Normalise Threshold to Oral Stimulation

### Gag reflex

To stimulate a hypo-active gag reflex.

*The therapist stimulates the gag reflex by touching briefly the soft palate with a cotton bud.*

NOTE
This technique will only rarely be necessary as the stimulating techniques above will usually result in a more normal threshold.

CHECK
Do not persist once gag reflex is present, as it is most unpleasant for the patient once the reflex is established.

### Hypersensitive Mouth

*Firm digital pressure starting in the least sensitive area and working towards the most sensitive area, that is, from lips to gums to anterior third of tongue.*

NOTE
Techniques to normalise threshold are followed by the training of missing components.

## To Encourage Facial Movements

*Jaw held closed, patient tries a little smile while therapist indicates with her finger the direction in which movement should occur (Fig. 3.5).*

INSTRUCTIONS
'Can you smile? Try to use this side of your face—no, keep the other side relaxed.'

CHECK
Lips should be gently closed.
Do not allow overactivity of intact side.

NOTE
Do not give bilateral facial exercises, as these will increase the tendency towards overactivity of the intact side. The patient needs not only to activate the muscles on the affected side, but also to decrease activity on the intact side.

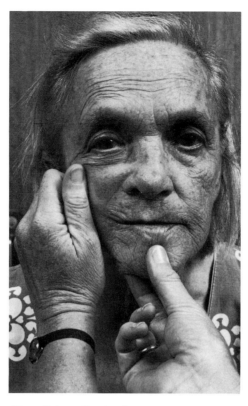

**Fig. 3.5** *The therapist indicates the direction of movement while patient attempts to smile without overactivity of the intact side.*

### To Improve Breathing Control

NOTE

Some patients have difficulty with breathing control following stroke, either because respirations are too shallow, or because they are impersistent. Shallow respirations leave the patient prone to respiratory infections and do not allow effective oxygenation. Motor impersistence interferes with vocalisation. The following technique is useful in both cases.

*Patient sits with trunk inclined forward, arms resting on a table. He practises deep breathing with the emphasis on expiration. Therapist gives overpressure and vibrations on lower third of rib cage on expiration. This can be combined with the patient making a sound on expiration. The patient can also experiment with varying the sound. This provides useful auditory feedback. This technique is also useful as preparation for speech therapy.*

INSTRUCTIONS
'Take a deep breath. Breathe right out gently, I'll help you.'
'Now say "ah", "m" as you breath out.'

CHECK
Make sure patient does not feel embarrassed if he is expected to do this in an open treatment area.

Another method of improving breathing control enables the patient to regain control over tongue and soft palate. It is also useful for helping the patient to gain control over outbursts of crying.

*Patient holds air in his cheeks while he breathes in and out through his nose in a relaxed manner.*

INSTRUCTIONS
'Hold some air in your cheeks.'
'Keep your lips closed and breathe quietly through your nose.'

CHECK
Make sure patient keeps air in cheeks—this means he has closed off the posterior oral cavity.

## To Improve Control over Emotional Outbursts

Treatment consists of training to improve control over oral musculature and ventilation as well as helping the patient to modify his behaviour. He should be reassured that the therapist understands the problem and that there are strategies for overcoming it. The therapist's manner should be calm and firm as she takes the appropriate action to help him modify his behaviour.

*Whenever the patient looks as if he is about to cry.*

INSTRUCTIONS
'Take a deep breath.'
'Now just breathe quietly through your nose if possible.'

NOTE
The patient will learn to use this strategy when necessary.

*If the patient has lost control and is actually crying, therapist holds jaw closed gently.*

INSTRUCTION
'Take a deep breath and stop crying.'
When patient gains control, 'Good'.

### STEPS 3 AND 4    PRACTICE OF ORO-FACIAL FUNCTION AND TRANSFERENCE OF LEARNING INTO DAILY LIFE

Liquid is more easily aspirated than food, hence the patient will gain some confidence in his ability to swallow without choking if he practises swallowing solids before he attempts liquids. Food should be palatable, consist of a variety of textures and initially should be of the consistency of mashed potatoes. Bosma[2] comments that thickened food is usually handled with relative safety. Pureed food or food which goes sloppy in the mouth will not provide the stimulus needed for regaining normal oral function and may be easily aspirated.

The patient should also be given chewable food. If he has difficulty with chewing, he may find it easier if the therapist holds his jaw lightly closed.

The therapist should assist the patient with his first few meals. She should use the techniques described earlier depending on her analysis of any difficulty he has while eating. She should give the relevant parts of the oro-facial section of the Programme just before at least one meal a day while such intervention is necessary. Nurses and relatives should be taught to reinforce this. The patient should sit up at a table to eat and mealtimes should be organised so that they are pleasurable and social occasions.

During all the sections of this Programme, the therapist constantly monitors the patient's facial posture while he concentrates on various activities. She indicates to him when his lips and jaws are open and reminds him to keep them closed, she stimulates the cheek to encourage activity and discourages overactivity of the intact side. The therapist uses her own facial expression in order to encourage the more passive person to respond.

The patient who is having difficulty keeping his false teeth in place because of diminished sensory awareness should be shown how to rub his gums briskly, and he should do this himself prior to putting his teeth in.

The strategy for gaining control over emotional outbursts (described on p. 72) should be explained to nursing staff and relatives, so they will be able to remind the patient to use it when necessary. Consistency in this will prevent emotional outbursts from becoming habitual.

Improved breathing control, a more active mobile tongue and the ability to control a prolonged expiration will enable the speech pathologist to improve verbal communication skills in the patient who is dysarthric.

Improved oro-facial control and appearance will help the patient regain confidence in personal interactions with staff, relatives and other people. He should be encouraged to socialise and try out his new abilities.

The oro-facial problems described are quickly overcome if the correct therapy is instituted within the first few days and if the therapist ensures the opportunity for consistent practice. If at this early stage the patient dribbles food or saliva, he should have extra time spent on techniques to improve tongue function and swallowing. This will ensure that the normal swallow mechanism becomes quickly retrained and wiping of the mouth does not become the habitual response to the collection of saliva. The patient needs to understand the importance of lip and jaw closure to a more effective swallow. Nose breathing may need to be stressed throughout therapy sessions with patients who have not yet re-established habitual closure of the lip and jaw.

## REFERENCES

1. Larsen G. J. (1972). Rehabilitation for dysphagia paralytica. *J. Speech Dis;* **37**:187–94.
2. Bosma J. F. (1957). Deglutition: pharyngeal stage. *Physiol. Rev;* **37**:275.
3. Williams P. L. and Warwick R., eds (1980). *Gray's Anatomy*, 36th edn. London: Churchill Livingstone.
4. Fisher M. (1956). Left hemiplegia and motor impersistence. *J. nerv. ment. Dis;* **123**:201–18.
5. Ben-Yishay Y., Diller L., Gerstman L. and Haas A. (1968). The relationship between impersistence, intellectual function and outcome of rehabilitation in patients with left hemiplegia. *Neurology;* **18**:852–61.
6. Mueller H. (1971). Personal communication.
7. Kydd W. L. and Toda J. (1962). Tongue pressure exerted on the hard palate during swallowing. *J. Amer. dent. Ass;* **65**:319–30.

# 4

## *Sitting up from supine*

Most people, when they sit up over the side of the bed, go from supine to sitting up, use the hands for leverage and swing the legs over the side of the bed. The elderly often roll to one side first, use one hand to push themselves up, then swing the legs over the side. In the early stages following stroke, it is practical and more effective for the patient to be helped to roll on to his intact side and to sit up from this position. There are two reasons for this: (i) it avoids the unrestrained use of the intact arm which results when the patient tries to pull himself up from supine into sitting, and (ii) it is a quick and easy way for the patient to get up with minimal help from another person.

At this early stage, attempts at learning to move again are concentrated on motor activities in sitting and standing. However, rather than bodily lifting the patient into sitting, the therapist gives him the opportunity to recall the movements required and to relearn the essential parts of the sequence. He is thus assisted to participate as much as he can in sitting up without undue effort and overuse of the intact side. If the therapist applies leverage correctly at his shoulder and pelvis and if the patient lifts his own head laterally, sitting up requires very little effort from either therapist or patient. It is recommended that only a minimum period of time be spent on this section, as it is more important that the patient spends his therapy session practising movement in sitting and standing.

### DESCRIPTION OF NORMAL FUNCTION

In rolling on to one side, say the right, the head flexes and rotates towards the right, the left arm flexes at the shoulder, the shoulder girdle protracts and the body is rotated towards the right. This results in a shift of weight to the right side. The left leg flexes at the hip and knee and the foot pushes into the bed to provide leverage and to roll the body over. The underneath leg is usually flexed at the hip and knee, and the hips are shifted backwards in order to give a more stable base of support (Fig. 4.1).

In order to sit up over the side of the bed from the side-lying position, the neck and trunk flex laterally, the lower arm abducts into the bed to provide leverage and the legs are lowered over the side of the bed (Fig. 4.2).

NOTE

Rolling over is often given excessive emphasis in rehabilitation.[1,2] In the early stages, the patient is relatively helpless in supine and it is better for the therapist to assist him on to his side and to concentrate his practice sessions on other activities which are more stimulating as well as being more relevant for a person who should be spending his day out of bed.

ESSENTIAL COMPONENTS

*Rolling on to the side* (Fig. 4.1)

**Fig. 4.1** *Rolling on to the R. side.*

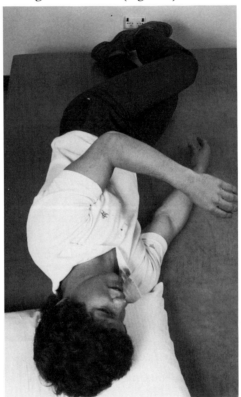

- Rotation and flexion of neck.

- Hip and knee flexion.

- Flexion of shoulder and protraction of shoulder girdle.

- Rotation within the trunk.

*Sitting up over side of bed* (Fig. 4.2)

- Lateral flexion of neck.

- Lateral flexion of trunk (abduction of the lower arm occurs as these two components are performed).

- Leg lowered over side of bed.

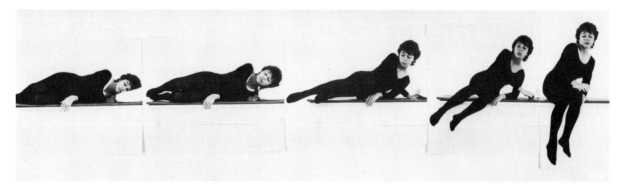

**STEP 1**     ANALYSIS OF SITTING UP FROM SUPINE

In **rolling on to the intact side**, the patient may demonstrate particular difficulty in:

- flexion of hip and knee on affected side
- flexion of shoulder and protraction of shoulder girdle.

These problems will result in:

- inappropriate compensatory movements of the intact side, e.g. he may try to wriggle or to pull himself over using his intact hand.

In addition:

- failure to move the affected arm passively across his body may indicate that he is neglecting the affected side.

**Fig. 4.2** *Sitting up over the side of the bed. Note the lateral flexion of neck and trunk.*

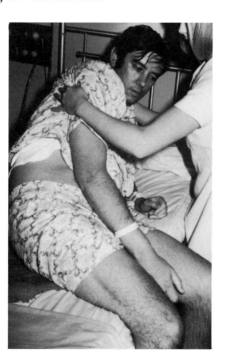

**Fig. 4.3** *This man is having difficulty laterally flexing his head and trunk. Note that his hips are insufficiently flexed, and that his weight is too far back.*

In **sitting up over the side of the bed**, the following problems may occur in compensation for the absence of essential components.

- Patient rotates neck and flexes it forward instead of flexing it laterally. This usually occurs because of poor lateral trunk movement (Fig. 4.3).

- Patient pulls with intact hand (at bedclothes or side of bed) instead of laterally flexing neck and trunk.

- Patient hooks intact leg under affected leg in order to get legs over side of bed. This will shift his weight back as he attempts to sit up.

### STEP 2      PRACTICE OF MISSING COMPONENTS

NOTE
Therapist assists patient on to his intact side. It is important that he does not have to struggle. The therapist encourages him to turn his head, assists him to bring his shoulder and arm forward, and to flex his hips and knees and, with one hand at his shoulder and the other at his pelvis, she rolls him on to his side. She may have to adjust his pelvis and legs in order to provide a stable base of support.

### To Stimulate Protraction of Shoulder Girdle for Rolling Over

*Lying on intact side, shoulder flexed forward at more than 90° with elbow extended, patient attempts to protract shoulder girdle with rotation of trunk forward (Fig. 4.4).*

INSTRUCTIONS
'Reach forward with your hand' or 'Reach towards me with your hand'.

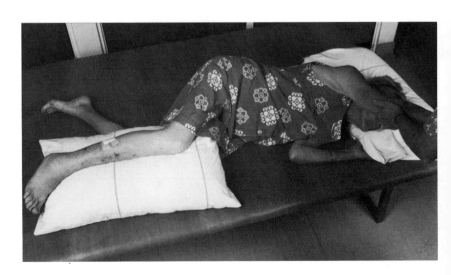

**Fig. 4.4(a)** *This woman is reaching forward with her arm. Note that the arm is held in some external rotation.*

CHECK

Do not pull on arm (as this will damage soft tissues around shoulder).
Do not allow patient to pull back at completion of movement. There is no
need to emphasise the return of movement.
Make sure wrist is extended.
Gleno-humeral joint must not be in internal rotation.
Do not resist movement.

Followed by:

*Half way between supine and side lying, pillow behind back, patient protracts
shoulder girdle with rotation of trunk as before. Patient this time must move
his upper trunk away from pillow (Fig. 4.4b).*

INSTRUCTIONS
'Reach towards me and roll on to your side.'

CHECK
As above.

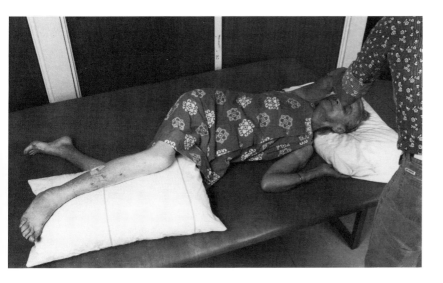

Fig. 4.4(b) *Now she is about to roll the top part of her body forward while reaching out with her arm. Therapist is guiding the direction of the movement.*

## To Stimulate Extension of Hip for Rolling on to the Side

NOTE
Although this is not necessarily an essential component of rolling on to the
side, it is included here as a means of encouraging the patient to use his
affected side to assist in the movement.

*Lying on intact side, knees flexed, patient attempts to extend his hip bringing
his pelvis forward. It may help him if he pushes through his heel. Therapist
passively moves pelvis backwards a few degrees in order for him to repeat the
movement (Fig. 4.5).*

INSTRUCTIONS
'Move your hip forward.'
'Push back gently with your heel.'

CHECK
Support the leg so it does not internally rotate or adduct, as this malalignment of the leg will interfere with the movement.

Followed by:

*Lying in supine, both hips and knees flexed, patient rolls on to his side. Therapist will need to hold his affected foot on the bed.*

NOTE
It is not necessary for the patient to have mastered rolling on to his side before he is assisted to sit up over the side of the bed.

**Fig. 4.5** *Lying on her side, this woman practises pushing down through the heel to bring her hip forward. Therapist is holding leg in correct alignment.*

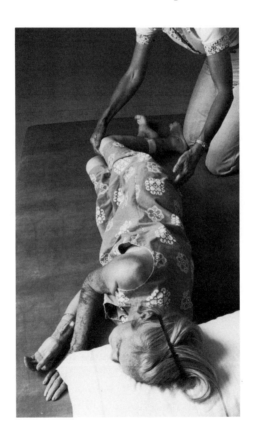

### To Stimulate Lateral Flexion of Neck

*Therapist assists patient to lift his head off the pillow and patient attempts to lower his head to the pillow, contracting his lateral flexors eccentrically. He then practises lifting his head sideways unaided (Fig. 4.6).*

INSTRUCTIONS

'Lower your head to the pillow.'
'Lift your head from the pillow.'

CHECK

Do not allow neck to rotate or flex forward.

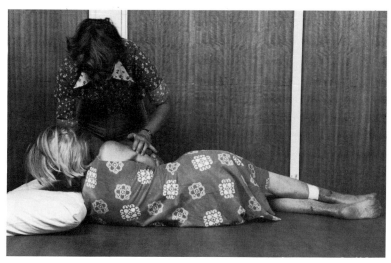

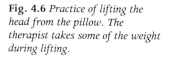
**Fig. 4.6** *Practice of lifting the head from the pillow. The therapist takes some of the weight during lifting.*

**STEP 3** PRACTICE OF SITTING UP FROM SIDE LYING

*Patient lifts his head laterally, while therapist, with one hand under the shoulder and the other pushing downwards on his pelvis, helps him to move up into the sitting position (Fig. 4.7a). Therapist may need to assist his legs over the side of the bed (Fig. 4.7b).*

INSTRUCTIONS

'Lift your head sideways.'
'Now, sit up and I'll help you.'

CHECK

Do not pull on patient's arm.
Continually remind him to keep his head moving sideways.
It may be necessary to move his legs over the side of bed before commencing the movement.
Do not let his weight go backwards.

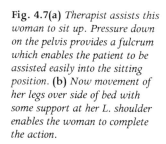
**Fig. 4.7(a)** *Therapist assists this woman to sit up. Pressure down on the pelvis provides a fulcrum which enables the patient to be assisted easily into the sitting position.* **(b)** *Now movement of her legs over side of bed with some support at her L. shoulder enables the woman to complete the action.*

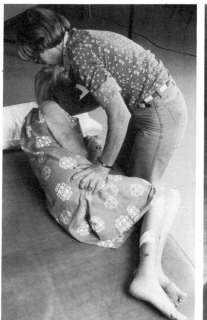

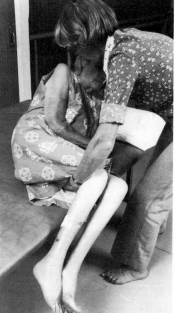

(a)                    (b)

## STEP 4    PRACTICE OF LYING DOWN

*From the sitting position, patient shifts his weight down sideways on to his intact forearm. Therapist reminds him to move his head laterally in the opposite direction as she lifts his legs up on to the bed.*
*Patient lowers himself down on to his side.*

INSTRUCTIONS
'Lower yourself on to your arm.'
'Lift your head sideways.'

CHECK
Do not pull on patient's arm.
Continually remind him to keep his head moving sideways.
Do not let his weight go backwards.

## STEP 5    TRANSFERENCE OF LEARNING INTO DAILY LIFE

The patient should not spend any more time in bed than is necessary for medical reasons (Fig. 4.8), nor should he spend any more time lying down than is necessary for sleeping or for the retraining of upper limb function in therapy sessions. The lying position reinforces drowsiness, confusion and feelings of helplessness, and provokes the symptoms of deprivation. Most patients early after stroke are helpless when in bed as their solitary attempts at movement are usually ineffectual. Movement, however, is necessary for its stimulating effect upon the reticular activating system. Early assumption of the erect position (i.e. sitting and standing) also has a stimulating effect upon the central nervous system, counteracts depression, enables the patient to regain control over bladder function and oral function, and encourages communication. The person who is virtually helpless in supine will usually be able to gain some control over sitting balance in one treatment session. It is therefore essential to assist him to sit up as soon as possible.

Nursing staff, therapists and relatives should follow the same procedure as given in this section when helping the patient out of bed in the morning and when helping him off the treatment couch, for as long as he needs assistance with this activity. The patient should not have a monkey ring suspended above his bed. Pulling down on a ring reinforces non-use of the affected side and emphasises overactivity of the intact upper limb.

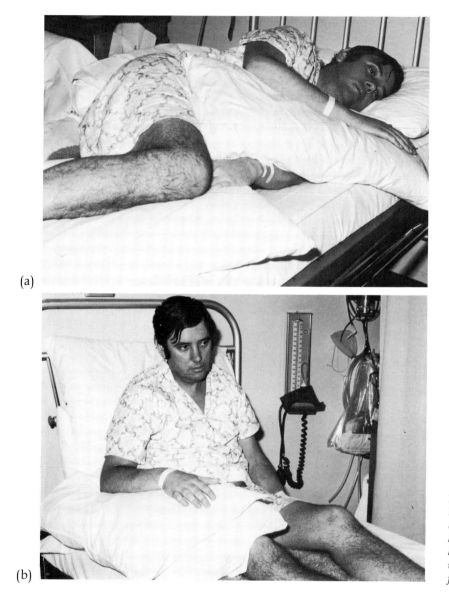

(a)

(b)

**Fig. 4.8(a)** *The patient confined to bed is positioned on his side with a device for keeping bedclothes off his feet.* **(b)** *While sitting in bed, he is positioned symmetrically with arm supported and hips flexed.*

## REFERENCES

1. Johnstone M. (1978). *Restoration of Motor Function in the Stroke Patient.* London: Churchill Livingstone.
2. Atkinson H. W. (1977). Principle of treatment (I & II). In *Neurology for Physiotherapists,* 2nd edn (Cash J., ed.) pp. 93–146 London: Faber & Faber.

# 5

# *Balanced sitting*

## DESCRIPTION OF NORMAL FUNCTION

The ability to be active in sitting requires that body alignment be appropriate and that the correct adjustments can be made to the changes in body alignment which occur with shifts in centre of gravity (i.e. with movement).

Balanced sitting involves the inability to sit without using undue muscular activity, to move about in sitting (Fig. 5.1), and to move in and out of the sitting position. Balance reactions consist of movements of the head, trunk, and limbs in response to any shift in the centre of gravity. They prevent a loss of balance. That is, when one body segment moves, the position of the centre of gravity alters, and this requires movement of other body segments in the opposite direction in order to rebalance the body. Actual movements may or may not be easily observable, depending on the degree of displacement. However, even small shifts in centre of gravity (i.e. even slight movements of the head, trunk or limbs) involve some motor activity. Normally, weight is taken through the arms or hand for protective support only when the centre of gravity has moved so far that balance is lost or is about to be lost.

**Fig. 5.1(a)** *and* **(b)***Reaching to floor for a cup. During this activity, which requires movement in both a lateral and an antero-posterior direction, complex adjustments are made to prevent loss of balance.*

(a)

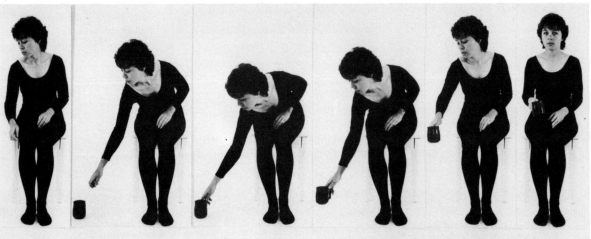

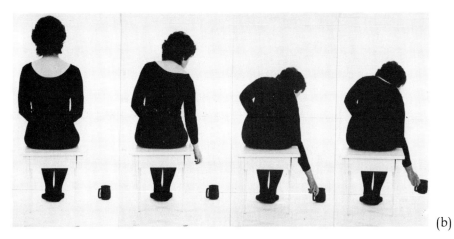

(b)

### ESSENTIALS OF SITTING ALIGNMENT

- Feet and knees close together.
- Symmetrical sitting.
- Flexion of hips with extension of trunk (i.e. shoulders over hips).
- Head balanced on level shoulders.

### ESSENTIAL COMPONENTS OF BALANCE REACTIONS

**Lateral shift in centre of gravity** (Fig. 5.2)

- Lateral flexion of neck.
- Lateral flexion of trunk, i.e. elevation of pelvis, depression of shoulder.

**Backward shift in centre of gravity** (Fig. 5.3)

- Forward flexion of neck.
- Forward flexion of trunk.

**Fig. 5.2** *Normal subject's response to displacement of centre of gravity laterally.*
**Fig. 5.3** *Normal subject's response to displacement of centre of gravity backwards.*

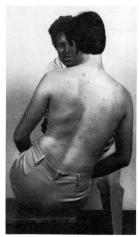

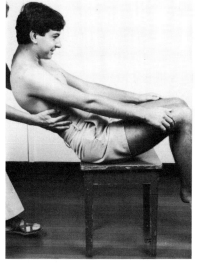

Fig. 5.2          Fig. 5.3

**STEP 1    ANALYSIS OF BALANCED SITTING**

Analysis of sitting consists of:

- observation of the patient's alignment in sitting
- testing of his ability to adjust to voluntary movement of limbs, trunk and head. Patient is asked, for example, to look behind him, to reach forward, sideways and backwards, to lift his intact leg, to pick up an object from the floor, to look at the ceiling.

The therapist notes any missing components (Figs. 5.4 to 5.6) and any abnormal compensatory responses and analyses the reasons for these problems. Below is a list of some compensatory responses which are commonly found in patients with poor sitting balance.

- Wide base of support, i.e. feet and/or knees apart (Fig. 5.5).
- Voluntary restriction of movement, i.e. patient holds himself stiffly and holds his breath.
- Patient shuffles feet instead of making adjustments with appropriate body segments.
- Protective support on hand or arm or grabbing for support with minimal movement. This patient may lose balance on any slight movement, even on taking a deep breath. He uses his hands to give himself a wider base and increase his stability.
- Patient leans forwards or backwards when weight should be shifting sideways. This means lateral flexion of the trunk is poor (Fig. 5.6).

**Fig 5.4** *This man has insufficient hip flexion. In compensation, his trunk and neck are flexed.*
**Fig. 5.5** *This man lacks lateral flexion of the trunk. In compensation, he has widened his base of support and is leaning forward.*
**Fig. 5.6** *This man lacks lateral flexion of his trunk. In compensation, he leans backwards.*

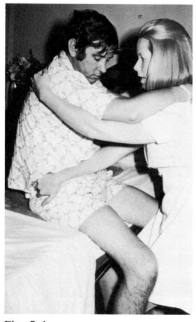

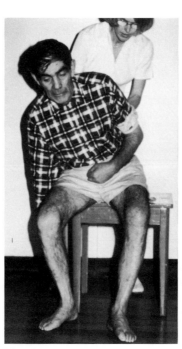

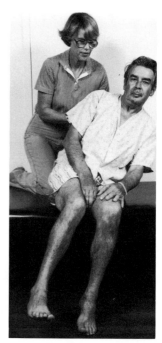

Fig. 5.4                    Fig. 5.5                    Fig. 5.6

**STEPS 2 AND 3    PRACTICE OF BALANCED SITTING**

The patient sits on a firm base with feet flat on the floor. Knees and feet must be a few inches apart. The therapist must ensure that the patient makes the necessary adjustments by moving his trunk and head, not by shuffling his feet, widening his base or wriggling about. The therapist must not hold him too much or he will not *need* to adjust. She must avoid the use of phrases such as 'Don't let me push you', 'Resist me' and 'I'm going to threaten your balance', as these will elicit an incorrect response. The patient should keep both hands resting in the lap when they are not required for the activity.

### To Stimulate Adjustments to Shifts in Centre of Gravity

NOTE
The first two techniques are useful for the patient, early after his stroke, who is frightened of moving. They take his attention away from the shift in his centre of gravity.

*In sitting, patient reaches forward, downwards towards floor and sideways, each time returning to the upright position. Therapist supports the affected arm while necessary (Fig. 5.7).*

INSTRUCTIONS
'Reach out and touch my hand.'
'Lift your head.'
'Now, sit up straight again.'
'Let's do it again—come on—see if you can reach a little further.'

CHECK
Make sure to correct head and trunk movement.
Direct patient's eyes towards a target.
Keep drawing patient's attention towards his affected side, making sure he has his weight on this side when appropriate.
Make sure he returns to the upright position slowly.

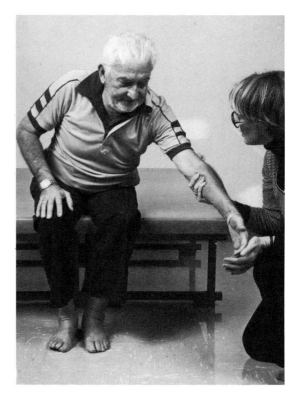

Fig. 5.7 *Therapist supports this man's affected arm while he reaches to touch her hand.*

*In sitting, hands in lap, patient turns head and trunk to look over his shoulder, returns to the mid position, repeats to the other side (Fig. 5.8).*

NOTE
This stimulates subtle adjustments. It shows the patient that he can move about, and enables him to regain a sense of balance.

INSTRUCTIONS
'Turn around and look behind you.'
'Turn your body as well as your head.'
'Don't lean back.'

CHECK
Do not allow him to rotate his legs to one side, i.e. make sure he keeps his knees facing forward.
Keep drawing patient's attention towards his affected side, making sure he has his weight on this side where appropriate.
Make sure he keeps his hands in his lap.

**Fig. 5.8** *Turning to look behind stimulates weight shift and gives him confidence in his ability to move in a balanced manner.*
**Fig. 5.9** *The patient practises taking weight through the affected arm and returning to the sitting position.*

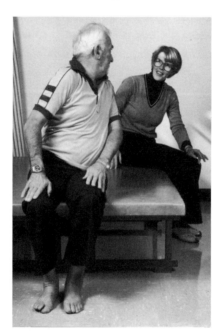

Fig. 5.8

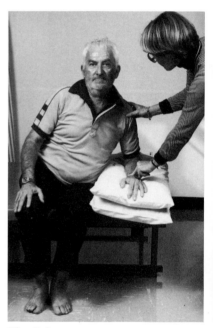

Fig. 5.9

*In sitting, therapist assists patient sideways to support himself on the forearm of his affected side on one or two pillows. Patient practises regaining the sitting position (Fig. 5.9).*

NOTE
This shows the patient how to control movement in sitting by introducing him to the trunk and head movements involved in balanced sitting.

INSTRUCTIONS
'I'm going to help you take some weight through this arm.'
'Now, sit up—lift your head first.'

CHECK
Do not allow him to lean back.
Make sure his shoulder is over his elbow, and his head flexes laterally.

*Therapist holds the patient's arm with shoulder girdle in some elevation and arm close to the trunk. She shifts his weight forward and sideways towards the affected side and encourages him to repeat the movement himself. Emphasis is on movement of the trunk and hips (Fig. 5.10).*

NOTE
This technique gives the patient the feeling of the correct body alignment during shifts of weight to the affected side. It also gives him the feeling of weight-bearing through the hand once his weight is on the affected side.

INSTRUCTION
'Bring your weight on to this side of your bottom.'

CHECK
Do not allow or encourage the patient to push down through his hand.
Do not allow him to pull his arm away or lean backwards when he is regaining the mid position.
Hold the elbow straight if necessary.
Wrist, elbow and shoulder should be in correct alignment.

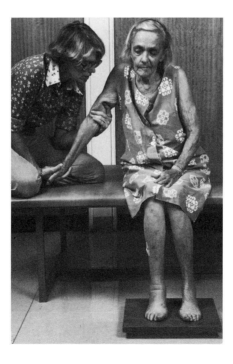

**Fig. 5.10** *Elevation of the shoulder girdle helps this woman to shift her weight actively on to the affected hip.*

*In sitting, the therapist holds the patient's arms extended and externally rotated behind him, with his shoulders elevated. She shifts him backwards so he takes weight through his hands (Fig. 5.11).*

NOTE
This technique encourages a symmetrical sitting position and controlled weight shift backwards as well as preventing contracture of the wrist and finger flexors.

INSTRUCTIONS
'Let me move you backwards. See if you can take weight through both hands.'

CHECK
Make sure patient's weight really does go backwards and that he is stimulated to take weight through both hands.
Do not allow elbow to bend.
His shoulders should be level.

**Fig. 5.11** *Therapist has shifted this woman's weight backwards with more emphasis on the L. side. Next, the patient will rest backwards for a few moments with her hands on the bed.*

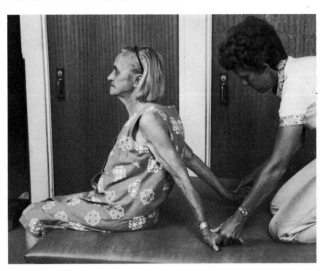

## To Stimulate Essential Aspects of Balanced Sitting Alignment

NOTE
If the patient cannot sit alone or if he is having difficulty extending his trunk, he may rest his arms/hands on the therapist's shoulders. However, the therapist must not move the patient passively or support him. He must make active responses himself. These techniques enable the patient and therapist to concentrate on specific components of balance reactions.

*Therapist teaches the patient to incline his trunk forward by flexing at the hips with head and trunk extended (Fig. 5.12a). This is followed by teaching him to move his trunk backwards by extending his hips with head and trunk flexed (Fig. 5.12b).*

(b)

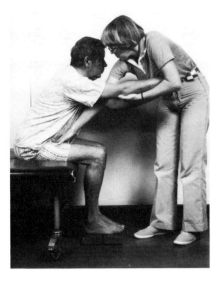
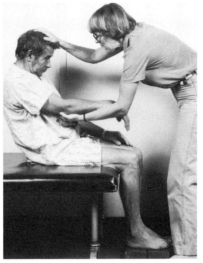

*Fig. 5.12(a) Therapist is indicating to this man that he must flex at his hips as he comes forward. (b) The therapist is reminding him to flex his head forward as he moves backwards.*

INSTRUCTIONS

'Bend forward at your hips. Keep your head up. Bring your head and shoulders forward.'
'Let your weight go back. Chin on to chest.'
'Now, sit up tall.'

CHECK

Make sure patient moves at hips and not at waist.
Make sure his weight is on both buttocks.
Encourage him to look at you as he moves forward.
Do not allow him to shuffle his feet or his bottom.
Do not pull on his arms.

*Therapist teaches the patient to shift his weight sideways by laterally flexing his head and trunk (i.e. elevating the pelvis). Return to the mid position and repeat to the other side (Fig. 5.13).*

*Fig. 5.13 Therapist is training this man to laterally flex his trunk, concentrating on lifting his L. hip from the bed. Elevation of his R. shoulder gives him the feeling of the alignment required. Note that he has been able to flex his head laterally to the L. and that his head position is satisfactory.*

INSTRUCTIONS

'Bring your weight over to this side of your bottom.'
'Keep your head up.'
'Lift your other hip.'
'Now, sit up again.'

CHECK

Do not allow him to widen his base by putting his knees and feet apart.
Make sure his weight does not go backwards—his shoulders should be over his hips.
Make sure his shoulder on the weight-bearing side is elevated as he shifts weight to this side.

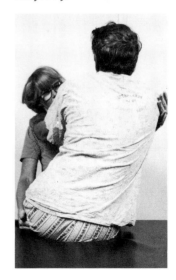

## To Increase Complexity

*Therapist holds the patient's flexed legs and rotates them from side to side, displacing his centre of gravity laterally (Fig. 5.14).*

NOTE
This is a way of progressing the former two techniques by requiring an automatic response.

INSTRUCTIONS
'See if you can balance when I move your legs.'

CHECK
Do not lift his legs too high or he will lose balance backwards.
Patient should not use his hands—they should remain in his lap.
Therapist should not move him so far that he loses balance.

The patient's ability to balance must be continually expanded by the addition to the Programme of more complex activities, such as:

*Sitting, reaching sideways and downwards to pick up an object from the floor.*

**Fig. 5.14** *Lifting the feet off the floor and rotating the legs displaces the centre of gravity and makes it necessary to use the trunk and head to preserve balance.*

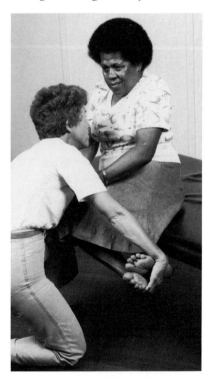

CHECK
Patient must go sideways and not forward.
Object must not be too close to chair.
Make sure patient returns to the upright position slowly.

*Sitting, reaching sideways to pick up an object from a table.*
*Sitting, reaching backwards to pick up an object (Fig. 5.15).*

NOTE
If the patient lacks sufficient hand control, he should try to touch the object.

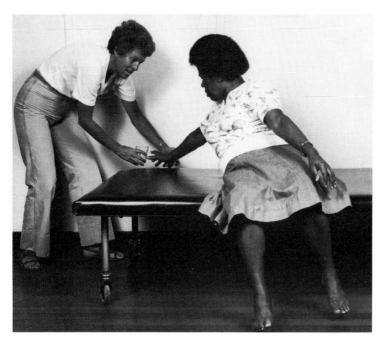

**Fig. 5.15** *Therapist moves glass to the outer limits of this R. hemiplegic person's range. She does not move it so far that the patient loses control and overbalances.*

### STEP 4    TRANSFERENCE OF LEARNING INTO DAILY LIFE

Throughout the day, whenever the patient is sitting, he should sit on a comfortable firm surface, with back supported, hips well back in chair, with shoulders level (a flaccid arm should be supported on pillows, p. 83). He should remember to shift his weight from one hip to the other from time to time. He may like to spend part of the day with his arms resting forward on a table. In this position, he will be able to read and do other activities.

The patient should be given his own check list with some major points to observe throughout the day—weight must be borne through both legs, the arm must be supported on a pillow or on a table.

# 6

# *Standing up and sitting down*

### DESCRIPTION OF NORMAL FUNCTION

Standing up and sitting down involves the placing of the feet and the shifting of the body in such a way that the centre of gravity is moved either forward or backwards with minimal expenditure of energy.

In **standing up**, one or both feet are moved backwards. This gives a base under the centre of gravity as it moves forward. Inclination of the extended trunk forward at the hips and movement of the body forward by dorsiflexion at the ankles brings the centre of gravity over the feet and enables the weight of the body to be shifted forward and upwards (Fig. 6.1). If the chair prevents the feet from moving far enough backwards, the trunk has to incline further forward or one has to move nearer the edge of the chair.

In **sitting down**, one normally checks the whereabouts of the chair by turning to look, feeling for the chair with the hand or feeling it against the back of the leg. The feet are positioned, the hips flex, inclining the trunk forward, so that, as the knees flex, the centre of gravity can be shifted

**Fig. 6.1(a)** *and* **(b)** *Standing up. Note the components and the sequence in which they occur.*

(a)

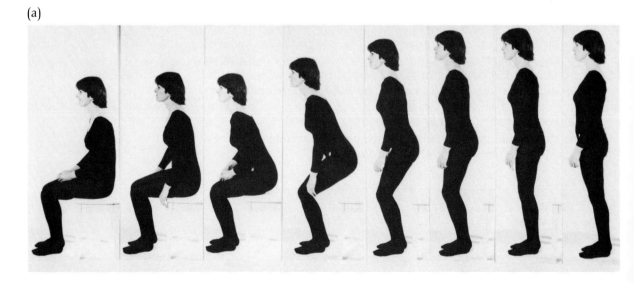

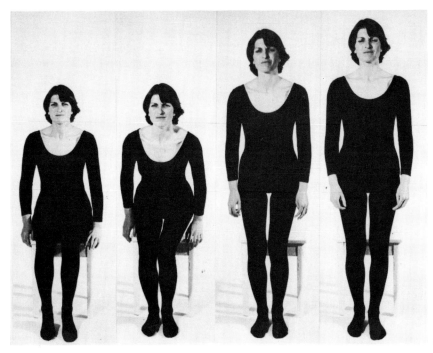

(b)

backwards without balance being lost. The body weight is lowered to the chair by a lengthening or eccentric contraction of the extensor muscles. It is the forward inclination of the trunk caused by flexion of the hips which enables the pelvis to move backwards and downwards towards the chair.

ESSENTIAL COMPONENTS

1. **Standing up.**
   - Foot placement.
   - Inclination of trunk forward by flexion at hips with extended neck and spine.
   - Extension of hips for final standing alignment.

2. **Sitting down.**
   - Inclination of trunk forward by flexion at hips with extended neck and spine.
   - Flexion of knees.

**STEP 1    ANALYSIS OF STANDING UP AND SITTING DOWN**

The therapist observes the patient's body alignment throughout the movement, or his attempts at the movement. The common problems are as follows.

- Weight is borne principally through the intact side (Fig. 6.2).

- Inability to shift centre of gravity sufficiently forward (Fig. 6.3).

- Patient tries to shift weight forward by flexing trunk and head instead of hips (Fig. 6.4) or by wriggling forward to the edge of the chair.

- Failure to place the affected foot ensures that the patient, who already has this tendency, will stand up and sit down with all weight taken through the intact side.

**Fig. 6.2** *This man's weight is principally on his intact R. side. His base of support is wide. His L. foot has not been placed back.*
**Fig. 6.3** *This man's centre of gravity is too far back. He did not initially incline his trunk far enough forward. He needs to practice this component.*

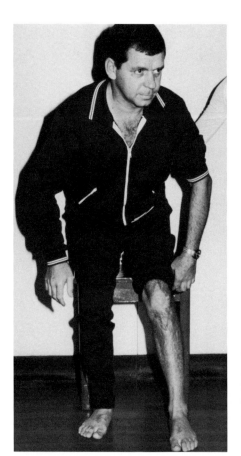

Fig. 6.2

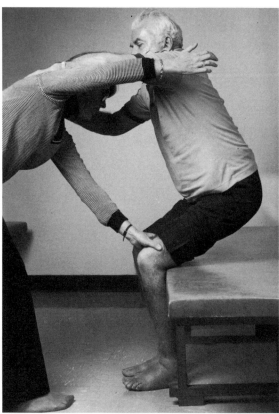

Fig. 6.3

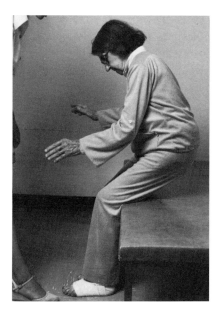

**Fig. 6.4** *This woman is sitting down. She is unable to incline her trunk sufficiently forward at her hips and flexes her head and upper trunk in compensation. Absence of flexion of the hips makes it impossible for her to stand up unaided.*

STEP 2      PRACTICE OF MISSING COMPONENTS

NOTE
The patient does not require good sitting balance in order to practise standing up. However, he does need good sitting alignment. How to achieve this is described in Balanced Sitting.

### To Stimulate Trunk Inclination Forward at Hips

*In sitting, feet flat on floor, patient practises inclining his trunk forward by flexing at the hips with the neck and trunk extended (see Fig. 5.12a).*

NOTE
Patient may rest his arms on the therapist's shoulders. Therapist elevates affected shoulder to preserve symmetrical body alignment and keep weight symmetrically distributed. Therapist will need to place patient's affected foot under the stool.

INSTRUCTIONS
'Bend forward at your hips. Keep your head up.'
'Bring your weight more to this side.'

CHECK
Avoid phrases such as 'Lean forward', 'Take your head to your toes', as these will encourage the patient to move incorrectly.
Do not stand too close to the patient as this will prevent the amount of hip flexion necessary to shift the centre of gravity forward.
Do not stand in a position which prevents the patient bearing weight through the affected side.

### STEP 3    PRACTICE OF STANDING UP AND SITTING DOWN

### Standing Up

If the patient is very weak, overweight, or unable to initiate movement, the therapist may need someone to assist her to stand him up (Fig. 6.5). A patient who has difficulty standing up will usually be able to gain some muscle control as he sits down, and practice of sitting down will eventually enable him to regain some control over the more difficult action of standing up. Practice of standing up may be facilitated by the use of a higher stool which eliminates some of the difficulty involved in initiating the activity.

*Fig. 6.5 This photograph illustrates how two people can assist a patient to stand. Although there may be two people needed, the emphasis is still on training the essential components.*

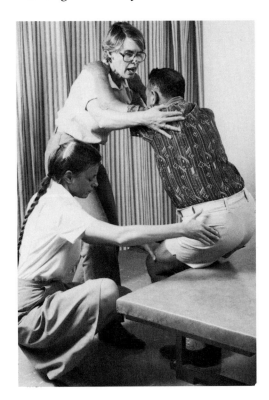

*When the patient's weight is sufficiently forward and symmetrical, he stands up. The therapist can keep his weight through the affected leg by pushing down through his knee towards his heel, then pulling the knee forward (Fig. 6.6).*

NOTE

Initially, it may be helpful for the patient to rest his arms on the therapist's shoulders as above. This is to enable the therapist to give him a little support and to encourage extension of the head and trunk. However, he must use his legs and not pull around the therapist's neck, link his hands around her neck or rest his weight too heavily upon her. In some cases (painful shoulder, short patient), it may be more satisfactory for the patient's hands to be at the therapist's waist (see Fig. 6.8).

INSTRUCTIONS
'Now stand up.'
When he is standing: 'Bring your hips forward/towards me.'

CHECK
Make sure weight is evenly distributed on both feet.
Do not wedge your knee against the patient's knee while he is standing up as this puts him off balance backwards.
Do not let the patient move to the edge of the chair when the chair is of the correct height and there is room for the feet to move back.
Do not extend the knee passively backwards when it should be shifting forward (Fig. 6.7).
Make sure the patient does as much movement as he can.
Make sure the trunk is inclined far enough forward and that the knees move forwards.

**Fig. 6.6** *Note the improved relationship between knee and ankle (compared with* **Fig. 6.3**)*, which indicates that the centre of gravity has moved forward. Now he can practise standing up and sitting down with weight through his affected (L.) leg.*
**Fig. 6.7** *The therapist demonstrates how, in an attempt to keep his knee straight, she can* **prevent** *a patient from extending his hips and bringing his centre of gravity forward.*

Fig. 6.6

Fig. 6.7

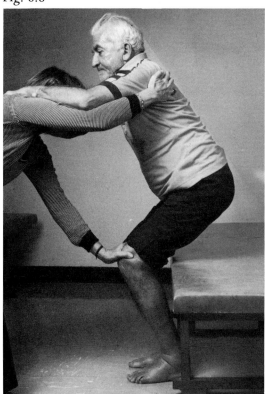

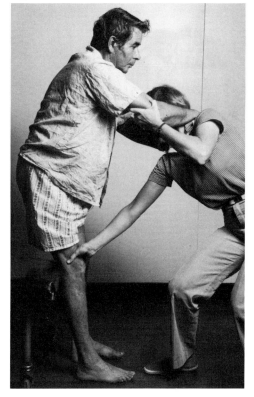

### Practice of Sitting Down

*The reverse of standing up (Fig. 6.8). The therapist may need to help the patient flex his knee and move it forward at the beginning of the movement. The therapist keeps the weight on the affected leg as he sits down by pushing down through his knee towards his heel.*

INSTRUCTIONS
'Move your bottom back and sit down.'

CHECK
Do not stand too close to the patient or hold his arms in such a way as to prevent him from inclining his trunk forward sufficiently. Do not prevent his knees from moving forwards.
Make sure weight is evenly distributed on both feet.

**Fig. 6.8** *Practice of sitting down. The therapist guides the movement to ensure that weight is taken through both feet. At this point the therapist is guiding the upper trunk forward and downward while the woman concentrates on moving her hips backwards and downwards.*

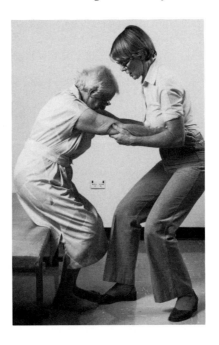

### To Increase Complexity

*When the patient gains some control over the movement he does not need his hands on the therapist's shoulders (Fig. 6.9).*

*Patient practises sitting to standing and standing to sitting, stopping in different parts of the range, changing direction and altering speed. The therapist directs these spatial and temporal variations.*

*Therapist asks patient to stand up and walk off to one side. Emphasis should be on walking to the affected side.*

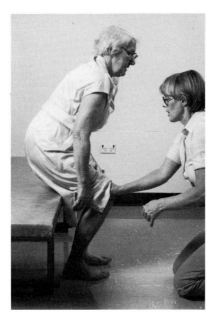

**Fig. 6.9** *The therapist helps this woman to maintain weight through her affected leg throughout the activity of standing up and sitting down by pressing down through the knee and pulling it forward.*

**STEP 4**      TRANSFERENCE OF LEARNING INTO DAILY LIFE

The patient should have the opportunity to practise this activity correctly with other members of the staff and relatives. He must not be allowed to pivot on his intact leg (Fig. 6.10) when moving (transferring) from bed to chair, from one chair to another, or from chair to lavatory, as this will encourage non-use of the affected side and prevent him from learning to stand up correctly. A major point in motor training is consistency of practice. There is no consistency if the patient practises one way in therapy and another way throughout the day. Consistency is not difficult to organise as it involves only a brief training session for close relatives, nursing staff and aides.

**Fig. 6.10** *Note how this man's weight and attention are directed towards his intact side when he uses his intact arm to push himself up into standing.*

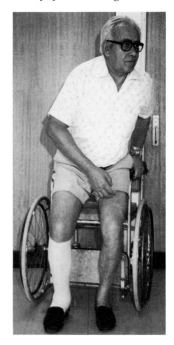

# 7

# *Balanced standing*

## DESCRIPTION OF NORMAL FUNCTION

The ability to be active in standing requires appropriate body alignment and that the correct adjustments can be made to the changes in body alignment which occur with shifts in centre of gravity (i.e. with movement).

### Balance

Balance in standing involves the ability to stand without using undue muscular activity, to move about in standing (including activities involving the head, trunk and limbs), to move in and out of the standing position and to walk, all without using the arms for support. Standing is not static but involves movement on a stationary base. The body continually sways, therefore there is a constant and accurately balanced movement of the centre of gravity to keep the line of gravity falling just in front of the ankles.

### Alignment

A well-aligned position requires less energy than a poorly aligned position. The most balanced position for standing requires that the feet be a few inches apart so that the legs are vertical. This gives the best base of support, not so large or so small that it introduces a diagonal force against the ground. The shoulders should be directly above the hips, hips extended, head and trunk erect. This normal alignment of body segments allows the person to move about and function effectively because he is well enough balanced to do so.

## ESSENTIALS OF STANDING ALIGNMENT

- Feet a few inches apart.
- Symmetrical weight-bearing.
- Extended hips.
- Extended knees.
- Hips over feet.
- Shoulders over hips.
- Head balanced on level shoulders.
- Erect trunk.

## ESSENTIAL COMPONENTS OF BALANCE REACTIONS

### Lateral shift in centre of gravity (Fig. 7.1).

- Lateral flexion of neck.
- Lateral flexion of trunk, i.e. elevation of pelvis, depression of shoulder.

**Fig. 7.1** *A normal subject's response to lateral shift in centre of gravity. Note in frames 2 and 3 that even a slight shift requires an adjustment of the body segments in the opposite direction.*

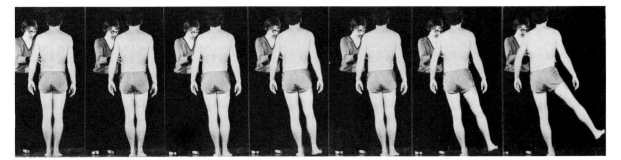

### Backwards shift in centre of gravity (Fig. 7.2)

- Extension of neck.
- Forward inclination of trunk at hips.
- Dorsiflexion of feet.

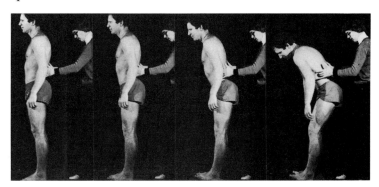

**Fig. 7.2** *A normal subject's response to backwards shift in centre of gravity.*

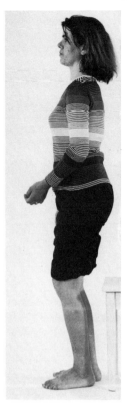

**Fig. 7.3** *This woman lacks hip and knee extension, i.e. her alignment is abnormal.*

**STEP 1    ANALYSIS OF BALANCED STANDING**

Analysis of standing consists of the following.

- Observation of the patient's alignment in standing (Fig. 7.3).

- Testing of his ability to adjust to voluntary movements of limbs, trunk and head. Patient is asked, for example, to look behind him, to reach forward, sideways and backwards, to stand on one leg, to pick up an object from the floor, to look up at the ceiling.

- Testing of his response to displacement of weight sideways and backwards (i.e. his balance or equilibrium reactions) with feet a few inches apart. Weight should be displaced at the waist so as not to interfere with the normal response.

The therapist notes any missing components (Figs. 7.4 to 7.7) and any abnormal compensatory responses and analyses the reason for these problems. Below is a list of some compensatory responses which are commonly found in patients with poor balance.

- Wide base of support, i.e. feet too far apart or one or both hips externally rotated (Fig. 7.5).

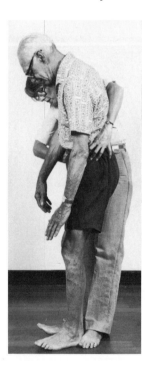

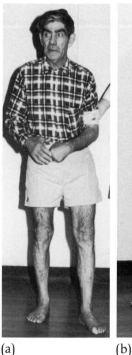

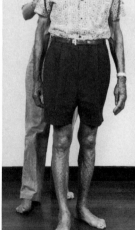

(a)                    (b)

**Fig. 7.4** *This man lacks sufficient flexion at the hips and dorsiflexion of his left foot when his centre of gravity is displaced backwards.*

**Fig. 7.5(a) and (b)** *These men both demonstrate a wide base of support. The man in* **(b)** *has given himself a wider base by externally rotating his L. leg.*

- Voluntary restriction of movement, i.e. patient holds himself stiffly and holds his breath.

- Patient shuffles feet instead of making adjustments with the appropriate body segments.

- Patient takes a step sideways or backwards as soon as centre of gravity moves. This means that balance is lost too soon (Fig. 7.6).

- Patient leans backwards when centre of gravity shifts sideways. This means that lateral flexion of the trunk is poor (Fig. 7.7).

- Use of arms, i.e. grabbing for support, holding arms out sideways or forward, on minimal shift of centre of gravity.

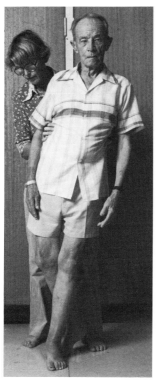 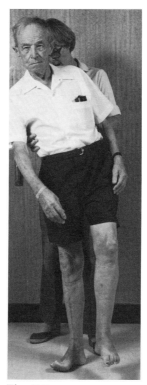

Fig. 7.6                Fig. 7.7

**Fig. 7.6** *This man is unable to make the appropriate adjustments to a lateral shift of weight to the L. He has taken a step with his R. leg to compensate for this.* **Fig. 7.7** *When his weight is shifted toward the R. side, he compensates for his lack of trunk lateral flexion by leaning backwards.*

**STEPS 2 AND 3    PRACTICE OF BALANCED STANDING**

NOTE

The relative importance of balance in different positions is often misunderstood. The patient does not need good balance in sitting before he is assisted to stand. There are differences in the relationships of body segments to each other and in the muscle action required in these two positions. He also does not need good balance in standing before he practises walking. Practice of walking and of the components of walking, with guidance from the therapist, will usually improve alignment and balance in standing.

All stroke patients, when they first stand up, are off balance. Many of them tend to drift to one side and backwards. Many patients react by shifting most of their weight on to the intact side. From the start, the patient must understand what is going wrong and how to correct it. He must know that the solution does not lie in holding on with his hands but in gaining control over his pelvis, legs and trunk. Similarly, the therapist must not panic and react by holding him up. If she resists this impulse and gives him the correct solution, for example 'Bring your hips forward' (with verbal feedback and manual guidance), he will quickly make an effective response himself.

It is important that the patient stands within the first few days and with weight on the affected side. This increases awareness of symmetry and bilaterality and enables him to commence training in balancing and walking skills. Balanced standing increases awareness of position in space and of body parts, which is particularly important for people with unilateral spatial neglect or diminished kinaesthetic sensation. Standing with weight through the affected leg in correct alignment may be one of the most important factors in preventing the development of unnecessary muscle activity in the limb and in training motor control.

Some patients, due to unilateral spatial neglect or to profound flaccidity, will find it easier to concentrate on gaining control over the pelvis, legs and trunk if the knee is controlled in a calico splint (p. 108). The limb load monitor* may also enable him to get the 'idea' of taking weight through his affected leg.

**To Stimulate Correct Standing Alignment**

**To Stimulate Hip Extension**

*Supine, leg over side of the bed, patient practises small-range hip extension (Fig. 7.8).*

---

*Krusen Research Center, Philadelphia, Pennsylvania.

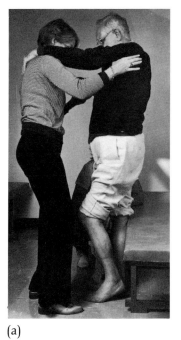

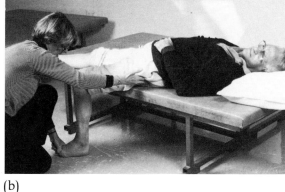

(a)  (b)

**Fig. 7.8(a)** *This man is unable to extend his hip and knee and therefore cannot take weight through the leg.* **(b)** *The therapist, having decided that lack of hip extension is the major missing component, trains the patient to contract his hip extensors.*

INSTRUCTIONS
'Push your heel gently down to the floor and lift your hip up a little.'
'Don't lift your hip too high.'

CHECK
Make sure the thigh is aligned correctly, i.e. that the hip is not abducted or internally rotated. Knee should be at a right angle.
If the knee tends to extend and the foot to plantarflex, hold the ankle and toes in dorsiflexion.
Make sure he does not move or tense up his intact side.
The objective is not to have the patient lift his hip from the bed but to contract his hip extensors.

Followed by:

*Patient stands with weight on both feet and hips extended (Fig. 7.9).*

NOTE
He is assisted to stand with weight on both feet as on p. 99. The improved alignment of the pelvis on the leg which results from the above technique usually enables the patient to develop some knee control.

INSTRUCTIONS
'Stand up.'
'Bring your hips towards me/forward.'
'Keep your weight over on this (affected) side.'

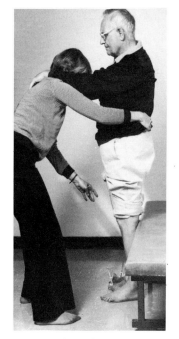

**Fig. 7.9** *After a few minutes practice of activating his hip extensors, he is able to stand with weight through the L. leg with the leg in normal alignment.*

*Patient takes a step forward with intact leg, then backwards.*

INSTRUCTION
'Keep your weight on this (affected) side.'
'Take a step forward.'
'Now backwards.'

CHECK
Do not allow hip on affected side to flex. It must extend as he steps forward with the intact leg.
Do not allow patient to shift pelvis too far laterally.
When patient steps forward, make sure he does not step to the side.

NOTE
If necessary, patient can rest his arms on the therapist's shoulders. This gives him a little support. His elbows should be extended and he should not hang on around the therapist's neck. Therapist should keep shoulders level.

### To Maintain Extension of the Knee

NOTE
Difficulty controlling the knee in the first few days is often a major factor in delaying standing activities. A calico splint (Fig. 7.10), put on in standing, enables the patient to bear weight through the affected leg without having to worry about his knee collapsing and allows him to practise controlling his hip (Fig. 7.11). He will be able to practise stepping forward with the intact leg, shifting his weight from side to side, and many of the balancing activities described below. Standing in the calico splint enables the patient to gain some muscular control of the knee, and the splint may only have to be worn for one or two sessions. An added advantage of the splint is to enable the therapist to stand a patient who

*Fig. 7.10(a) Calico splint made from a double layer of 80% duck, with two aluminium struts and Velcro straps. (b) Pattern for calico splint.*

(a)

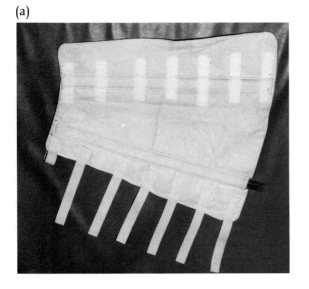

(b)

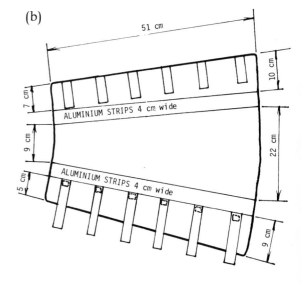

otherwise would be difficult to control. The person with unilateral spatial neglect, whose subjective midpoint has shifted towards the intact side, may find it impossible to bear weight through the affected leg without a calico splint.

Specific control over knee musculature is stimulated by the techniques on p. 127.

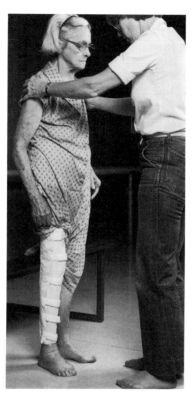

**Fig. 7.11** *This woman is practising shifting her weight on to the affected leg while controlling extension of the hip. The splint allows both her and the therapist to concentrate on the activity.*

## To Stimulate Adjustments to Shifts in Centre of Gravity

NOTE

The therapist must avoid the use of such phrases as 'Don't let me push you', 'Resist me' or 'I'm going to threaten your balance', as these will elicit an incorrect response (i.e. the patient will hold himself stiffly, widen his base, shuffle his feet). She must be careful not to hold the patient so much that no response from him is necessary. However, she should not allow him to overbalance. He should practise just within the limits of his ability, trying always to extend these limits. This means that the therapist must constantly monitor his body alignment. He must be actively discouraged from holding on or reaching out for support. He must be told how to use his pelvis and legs to balance, not his hands or arms; that is, he is taught what to do when he feels he is losing balance. If the patient tends to 'freeze' or stiffen, as he may do if he feels his balance is at risk, the therapist can use the first technique described below to deflect him from his rigid postural and mental 'set'. This technique shows him that he can move and still maintain his balance with only a little assistance.

*With feet a few inches apart or one in front of the other, the patient turns his head and trunk to look behind him, returns to the mid position, repeats to the other side (Fig. 7.12).*

INSTRUCTIONS
'Turn around and look behind you—turn your body as well as your head.'
'Don't move your feet.'

CHECK
Make sure standing alignment is preserved.
Do not allow patient to shift his feet. If necessary, place your foot next to his.

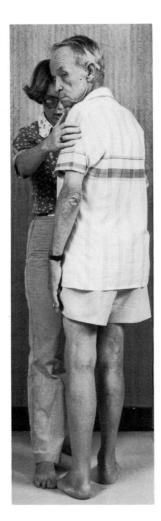

**Fig. 7.12** *With one foot in front of the other, the patient turns to look behind. Therapist monitors his alignment and prevents him from moving his feet.*

*With feet a few inches apart or one in front of the other, stimulation of controlled postural sway on a fixed base. Therapist rapidly displaces the patient's centre of gravity backwards and forward, and from side to side. (Alternate tapping.[1])*

NOTE

This technique is particularly useful for the patient who has virtually no balance in standing and who cannot stand alone. It can be done with the patient wearing a calico splint so he does not have to worry about his knee collapsing. This technique can also be used at various points throughout walking facilitation (see p. 137), but particularly at those stages of the walking cycle at which the person has poor balance (Fig. 7.13).

INSTRUCTIONS

'I'm just going to move you about a little. This will help you learn to balance again.' 'Don't hold yourself stiffly—let me move you.'

CHECK

Make sure to shift his centre of gravity—do not merely slap his trunk.
Do not push him off balance—he should not need to make gross adjustments.
Ensure correct body alignment, e.g. that his hips remain extended.
Do not allow him to shift his feet.
Do not ask him to resist or allow him to hold himself stiffly.
With patient in walk standing, therapist must incorporate some lateral weight shift and not just move the patient backwards and forward.
Vary the timing so it does not become predictable.

**Fig. 7.13(a)** *This man walks with his feet wide apart because he cannot balance if he walks with a narrower base.*
**(b)** *Therapist stimulates antero-posterior balance with patient standing with a more normal base of support.* **(c)** *She also stimulates balance in a lateral direction.*

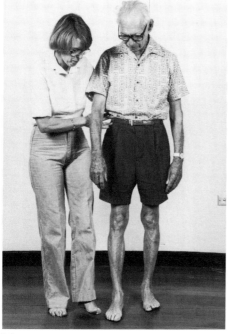
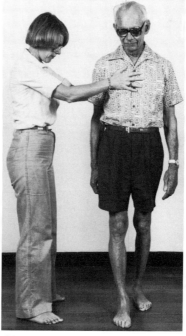
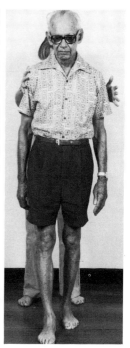

(a)                                   (b)                                   (c)

## To Stimulate Essential Aspects of Balanced Standing Alignment

*Therapist, moving him at the waist, displaces the patient's centre of gravity sideways, and teaches him to laterally flex his neck and/or his trunk. Patient returns to the mid position and centre of gravity is displaced to the other side (Fig. 7.14).*

**Fig. 7.14(a)** *Compare with Fig. 7.7. The therapist has shifted this man's weight to the intact (R.) side. He needs guidance to flex his head laterally to the L.* **(b)** *Here, the therapist has shifted his weight to the affected (L.) side. He has shifted too far to this side and has difficulty in making the correct responses.* **(c)** *Further practice with a smaller shift in centre of gravity, plus guidance in the performance of the components, enables him to make a more normal response.*

INSTRUCTIONS

'I'm going to move your weight sideways. See if you can keep from falling over.'
'Keep your head up.'
'Bend sideways at your waist—lift your hip up sideways.'
'Do not hold yourself stiffly, let me move you.'

CHECK

Do not shift his weight too far and push him off balance.
Make sure the weight-bearing hip remains extended.
Do not allow him to shuffle or take little steps.
Do not prod him at the shoulder.

(a)

(b)

(c)

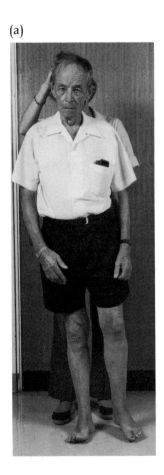
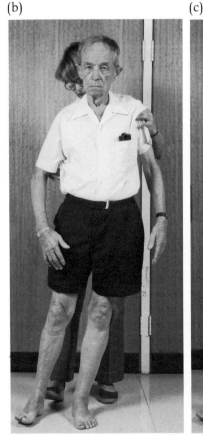
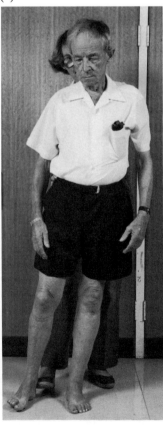

*Therapist, moving him at the waist, displaces the patient's centre of gravity backwards, encouraging flexion forward at the hips and dorsiflexion of the feet (Fig. 7.15).*

INSTRUCTIONS

'I'm going to move your weight backwards. See if you can keep from falling over.'
'Bend forward at your hips. Lift your toes up.'

CHECK

Make sure weight is on both feet.
Do not allow him to shuffle or take little steps. If necessary, block his feet with your foot.
Make sure he flexes at the hips.

NOTE

If the patient continues to have difficulty with foot dorsiflexion when his centre of gravity is shifted backwards, dorsiflexion can usually be successfully retrained by the following technique.

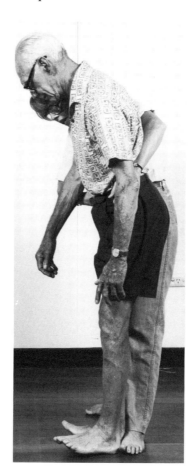

**Fig. 7.15** *Compare with Fig. 7.4. With practice of hip flexion and foot dorsiflexion in response to small shifts in centre of gravity backwards, this man is now able to make a more normal response.*

*Patient stands with back against a wall, feet a few inches away from it. Therapist holds his arms out in front with hands together. She places the patient's abducted thumbs between her thumb and index finger in a handshake grasp. The patient moves his hips away from the wall, therapist giving either slight resistance or assistance to guide the movement and ensure that his weight remains backwards. During the backwards and forward movement, the therapist looks for the point at which dorsiflexor activity is elicited and then confines the patient's movements around this point (Fig. 7.16).*

INSTRUCTIONS

'Bring your bottom away from the wall.'

'There, see how you are lifting your (affected) foot up a little. Try to lift it up a little more.'

CHECK

Do not allow patient to pull with his arms. He should move away from the wall with extended elbows.

Make sure his weight is evenly distributed.

Ensure that his knees do not flex.

Weight must stay back throughout.

**Fig. 7.16(a)** *When weight is displaced backwards, this man does not dorsiflex his L. foot.* **(b)** *and* **(c)** *The therapist is experimenting to find the point at which maximum dorsiflexion can be elicited.*

(a)

(b)

(c)

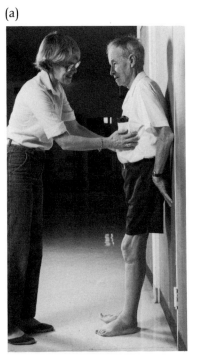
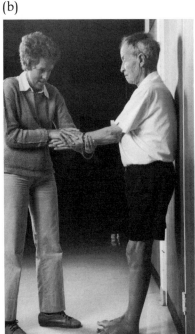
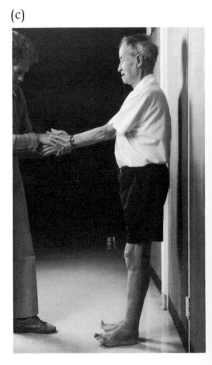

## To Stimulate Protective Support through the Arm

NOTE
This response involves weight-bearing through the arm and occurs when the centre of gravity falls so far outside the base of support that balance can no longer be maintained by adjustments of body segments. It is not an immediate response to shifts of weight but occurs only when balance is actually lost or is about to be lost; therefore, it is only retrained in this context. The technique below can only be attempted when the patient has some muscle activity in the shoulder, elbow and wrist.

*Patient stands at a suitable distance from a wall. Therapist gently pushes him off balance to stimulate protective support through the arm forward, backwards and sideways (Fig. 7.17).*

INSTRUCTIONS
'I'm going to put you off balance—use your hands when you want to.'

CHECK
Therapist may need to assist affected arm into correct position.

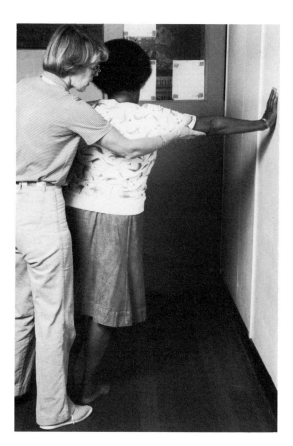

**Fig. 7.17** *Stimulation of protective support sideways. Therapist needs to assist the patient's arm into the fully abducted position.*

## To Increase Complexity

The patient's ability to balance must be continually expanded by the addition to the Programme of more complex activities. These may vary from talking to the therapist while standing with a narrow base to bimanual activities in standing, such as the following.

*Catching a ball thrown in such a way as to stimulate him to reach sideways, forward and downwards, and to step out to catch it.*

*Picking up from the floor different sized objects with the one hand and/or bimanually.*

*Practice of the components of walking in the standing position (p. 130) and walking itself improves balance, and variety and complexity can be added by having the patient stop when asked, change direction, step over objects.*

### STEP 4    TRANSFERENCE OF LEARNING INTO DAILY LIFE

From the first time the patient stands up, and this includes when he is assisted to get out of bed to sit on a chair, whoever is with him should make sure that he has practice of standing, but only with his body segments aligned correctly and with weight borne on the affected side. The patient himself should understand that these are the components he must practise whenever he gets the opportunity, and he could be given a check list of these major points so that he can monitor his own performance. Both he and the person helping him must make sure he does not pivot on the intact side when transferring from bed to chair. He should stand up with guidance (as described on p. 99), and he will learn more quickly to support his weight on the affected leg if he stands up in this way.

As soon as possible, the patient should spend short periods during the day standing at a bench. The limb load monitor can be used to ensure that he supports some of his weight on the affected leg. The bench should be of an appropriate height to encourage hip extension.

### REFERENCES

1. Bobath K. and Bobath B. (1964). The facilitation of normal postural reactions and movements in the treatment of cerebral palsy. *Physiotherapy*; **50**: 246–59.

# 8

# *Walking*

### DESCRIPTION OF NORMAL MOVEMENT

Normal walking in an adult involves a movement of the centre of gravity through space in such a way as to require the least possible expenditure of energy.[1] It requires little muscle activity and is rhythmical and symmetrical in nature. Adults walking normally take approximately 100 steps per minute.[2] Walking is a complex function and, although there have been many biomechanical and electromyographical studies,[3–5] there is as yet no complete picture of what is involved. Several gait laboratories are attempting to establish normative data.

Electromyographical studies indicate that, during the walking cycle, muscles act only over brief periods,[3,6,7] the limbs being carried forward to a large extent by their own momentum. Muscular activity is said to be involved more in deceleration than in actual progression. For example, the major action of the pretibial extensor group does not occur to lift the foot but at a point immediately after heel contact to decelerate the foot.[2,6] Gluteus maximus acts briefly following heel contact, then again at the end of the stance phase. The hamstrings contract and reach a peak of activity

**Fig. 8.1** *The normal sequence of walking.*

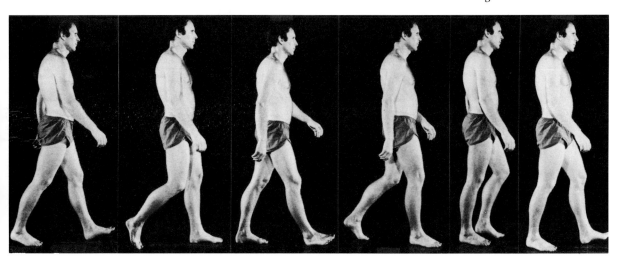

just after heel strike, and then again at the end of stance phase. The quadriceps also show their major activity before and at heel strike to decelerate the leg and then to absorb the impact by allowing a controlled flexion just after heel strike. Rectus femoris acts to control the pre-swing phase yield of the knee.[7]

Energy storage and recovery are efficient in normal walking because of the precise relationship between muscle contraction and displacement of body and limb segments and the brief periods during which muscles are active.[6] These factors also ensure that walking is rhythmical, with a natural cadence.

For the purposes of description, walking can be divided into stance (support) phase and swing phase (Fig. 8.1).

## Stance Phase

This phase, which begins with heel strike, is characterised by plantarflexion then dorsiflexion of the ankle; flexion of the knee (the 'yield' of the knee) which is followed by extension, with flexion occurring at the end of the phase; and extension of the hip which is continuous throughout the phase. These components enable the centre of gravity to be translated forward. Extension of the hip at the end of the stance phase

**Fig. 8.2** *Normal walking. Note (i) the very small lateral shift in the centre of gravity; (ii) the narrow base of support; (iii) the head and trunk adjustments to the lateral shifts.*

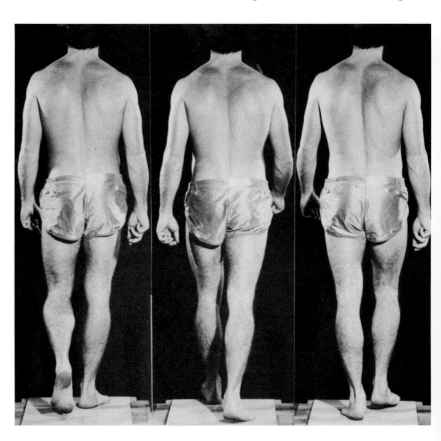

appears to be essential for the initiation of the swing phase of that leg, allowing the switch to be made from one phase to the other.[8] The flexion–extension–flexion of the knee gives walking its smoothness. As weight is shifted forward and laterally, the pelvis is prevented from dropping down or 'listing' on the opposite side more than the normal few degrees by contraction of the hip abductors of the supporting leg and the trunk lateral flexors of the non weight-bearing side (Fig. 8.2). That is, the hip joint of the swing leg is never given the elevation of the hip of the stance leg. The knee of the swing leg must therefore continue its flexion in order to 'shorten' the leg and enable it to swing through.[6] The contraction of the hip abductors of the standing leg also serves to control the amount of pelvic shift sideways, which is minimal and only as much as is necessary to shift the centre of gravity sufficiently laterally to allow the opposite leg to swing through. Excessive lateral displacement of the centre of gravity is also corrected by the presence of the tibio-femoral angle; that is, the abduction of the tibia relative to the femur which occurs when the knee is extended and the femur is adducting at the hip.[6]

## Swing Phase

Early flexion of the knee at the beginning of swing phase decreases the moment of inertia of the lower limb, which in turn decreases the amount of hip flexor activity required.[1] The knee has virtually completed its flexion motion by the time the hip flexes and this combined hip and knee flexion shortens the leg and allows the swing foot to clear the ground following toe-off. The early swing phase is thus characterised by hip flexion, the completion of knee flexion and dorsiflexion of the ankle. The final period consists of knee extension prior to heel strike, and ankle dorsiflexion which terminates immediately following heel strike.

### Shift in Centre of Gravity

The shift of the centre of gravity forward is accomplished by shift of the body weight as a whole forward by movement at the ankle and hip. The stability of the body throughout walking is related to the width of the base of support. Although a position with feet a few inches apart is normal in standing, this foot position would involve an excessive lateral horizontal shift of the pelvis if carried through to walking. Instead, the feet move directly forward from a position close together (Fig. 8.2). This limits the amount of lateral shift to a minimum while at the same time giving stability. The shift in centre of gravity necessitates compensatory adjustments within the trunk and neck in order to preserve balance. This requirement is minimised during average walking, but becomes more necessary if speed is decreased. Walking too slowly not only requires more balance but it also causes variations in the person's usual walking pattern. Less postural adjustment is involved in fast walking.

In normal walking, rotation of the pelvis occurs in a horizontal plane, but the magnitude of this rotation is small (4° on either side of the central axis),[1] its maximum excursion occurring at heel strike. This pelvic rotation is counteracted by thoracic rotation. In their study, Murray *et al.*[9] found an absence of pelvic rotation in some of their subjects, and a significant positive correlation between stride length and rotation. Although Saunders *et al.*[1] listed pelvic rotation as a major determinant of walking, Murray and his co-workers suggest that pelvic and thoracic rotation may not be essential components of smooth walking.

Since the pelvis is a rigid structure, rotation takes place at the hip joints and in the joints of the spine. The hip joint rotates internally during its swing phase until the position of full weight-bearing during stance phase is achieved, when there is a reversal into external rotation.[6]

Sagittal rotation (anterior and posterior pelvic tilting) occurs through a mean excursion of 3°, with maximum anterior tilt occurring just before heel strike and maximum posterior tilt early in stance phase.[9]

**Arm swing** during walking is relaxed and counteracts the tendency of the trunk to rotate away from the supporting leg. For example, as the right leg swings forward, the pelvis tends to rotate towards the left side. This is counteracted by a forward movement of the left shoulder with an associated arm swing.

ESSENTIAL COMPONENTS OF WALKING (Figs. 8.1 to 8.3)

**Stance Phase**

- Extension of the hip throughout.

- Lateral horizontal shift of the pelvis and trunk (normally approximately 4–5 cm (1·5–2 in) in total.

- Flexion of the knee (approximately 15°) initiated on heel strike, followed by extension, then flexion prior to toe-off.

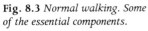

**Fig. 8.3** *Normal walking. Some of the essential components.*

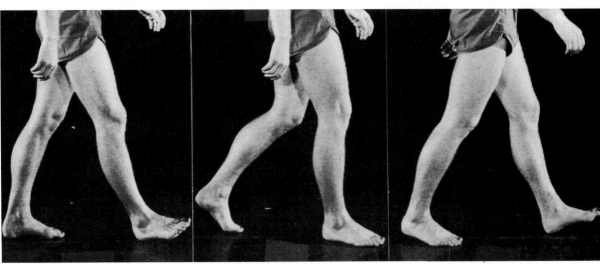

## Swing Phase

- Flexion of the knee.

- Lateral pelvic tilt downwards (approximately 5°) in the horizontal plane at toe-off.

- Flexion of the hip.

- Rotation of the pelvis forward on the side of the swinging leg (3–4° on either side of the central axis).*

- Extension of the knee plus dorsiflexion of the ankle immediately prior to heel strike.

The above components are the major determinants or biomechanical necessities of walking.

## Walking Backwards

Weight is not shifted backwards **during** swing phase in the same manner as it is shifted in walking forward. A new base is provided **before** weight is shifted because of the inherent instability of the activity. During swing phase, the hip and knee flex, then the hip extends a short distance with the knee held in flexion (Fig. 8.4) until the toes touch the ground. Only then is weight shifted backwards with further extension of the supporting hip and extension of the knee. Walking backwards is slower than walking forward, there are fewer visual cues and step length is shorter. Electromyographical studies indicate that muscles are more active than in forward walking,[10] which may be due to the relative lack of momentum in carrying the leg backwards.

## Walking Up and Down Stairs

Walking up and down stairs is described in detail by Andriacchi and his co-workers.[11]

Walking up stairs involves similar movement components to level walking, but the ranges of movement at the joints involved and muscle activity required are different in some respects. For example, a larger range of hip and knee flexion is required. When the foot is placed on the step, there is a forward inclination of the body at the supporting ankle and a forward and upwards shift in the centre of gravity over the forward leg (Fig. 8.5a).

*This does not need to be specifically trained as normal rotation will occur once hip extensions and knee control during stance phase, and knee flexion during swing phase have been trained.

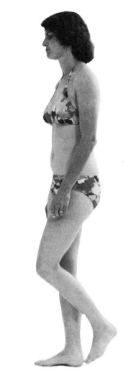

**Fig. 8.4** *Walking backwards. The L. knee is held in flexion while the hip is extending.*

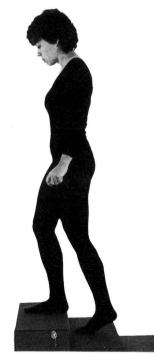

**Fig. 8.5a** *Walking up stairs.*

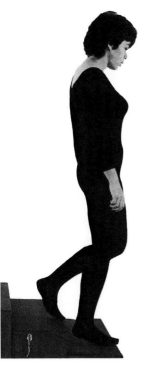

**Fig. 8.5b** *Walking down stairs.*

Walking down stairs has safety as its major consideration. Therefore, unlike both walking and walking up stairs, the centre of gravity is kept back over the supporting leg. The movement is performed by a controlled eccentric (lengthening) contraction of the hip and knee extensors of the supporting leg (Fig. 8.5b).

### STEP 1    ANALYSIS OF WALKING

The major problems found on analysis will be as follows.

**Stance phase of affected leg.**

- Lack of extension of hip (Fig. 8.6).

- Lack of controlled knee flexion (i.e. knee extensor activity) from 0–15° (Fig. 8.6).

- Excessive lateral horizontal shift of pelvis (Fig. 8.7).

- Excessive downwards pelvic tilt on the intact side associated with excessive lateral pelvic shift to the affected side (Fig. 8.7).

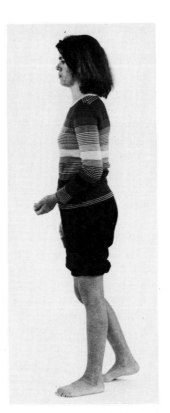

**Fig. 8.6** *This woman holds her knee in the fully extended position throughout stance phase because she lacks control over the quadriceps from 0–15°. Note also the lack of extension at the hip.*

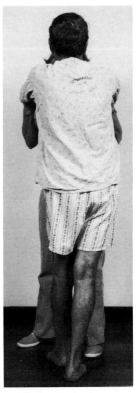

**Fig. 8.7** *This man has shifted his weight too far to his affected R. side. As a consequence, his pelvis has dropped down on the L. side.*

**Swing phase of affected leg.**

- Lack of knee flexion at toe-off (Figs. 8.8 and 8.9).

- Lack of hip flexion.

- Lack of knee extension plus ankle dorsiflexion on heel strike (Fig. 8.10).

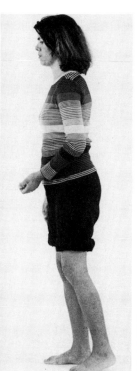 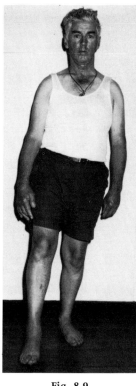 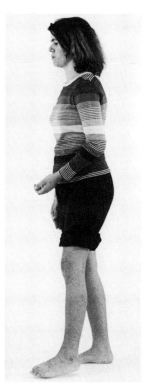

**Fig 8.8** *Swing phase of the affected leg. Note the lack of knee flexion at toe-off which is necessary to allow the foot to clear the ground.* **Fig. 8.9** *Note the elevation and backward tilt of the pelvis and abduction of hip in compensation for lack of knee flexion throughout the initial part of swing phase. Note the wide base.* **Fig. 8.10** *This woman lacks foot dorsiflexion and knee extension for heel strike. She has not translated her centre of gravity far enough forward at her R. hip.*

Fig. 8.8          Fig. 8.9          Fig. 8.10

In addition, the patient lacks the idea of the sequencing of components and of the rhythm and timing of walking.

Walking is a particularly complex activity and analysis of problems is difficult. However, analysis of the reasons why a patient cannot walk in the first few days after his stroke will usually indicate that he is unable to perform any of the essential components. It is important at this time that the therapist analyses the patient's problems correctly and makes the correct decisions about the components upon which training should concentrate. Below are some guidelines for the therapist to follow, particularly in the early period of training.

1. **Analysis and subsequent training always begin with the affected leg in stance phase**. It is essential that the patient acquire the

ability to bear weight through this leg in normal alignment with hip extension, controlled knee extension and the ability to shift the centre of gravity approximately 2·5 cm (1 in) laterally to the affected side. The patient will then be able to practise stepping forward with his intact leg, and once he can do this, analysis and training of the missing components of the swing phase of the affected leg can commence.

Although it may appear when the patient first stands up that his major difficulty is in initiating swing phase, it will be much easier to retrain the essential components in this phase once he has control of weight-bearing through the affected leg. There are probably several reasons for this. (a) Control of the pelvis on the leg is essential to the assumption and maintenance of a well-aligned position, as the pelvis provides a link between the supporting leg and the rest of the body. (b) Once some motor control is gained in stance phase, the muscles which are involved in the swing phase seem to be in a state of 'readiness'. (c) The hip flexors seem better able to swing the affected leg forward when this leg is positioned behind the intact leg, as the extended position of the hip initiates the pendular movement involved in swing phase. This is not the case from the standing position, when the hip flexors must work immediately against the full force of gravity. Flexion of the hip requires three times the amount of energy when knee flexion is absent[1] and hence the hesitancy seen at the start of swing phase if the patient attempts to set off with his affected leg first.

2. **Difficulty translating or shifting the centre of gravity laterally** in order to free the intact leg for swinging forward. Most patients shift their pelvis too far laterally and this results in a compensatory tilt of the pelvis downwards on the intact side (see Fig. 8.7). This excessive lateral shift is usually due to an unawareness of the normal extent of shift and to a difficulty contracting the ipsilateral hip abductors and contralateral trunk side flexors at the appropriate moment. It may result in part from lack of control over the last few degrees of knee extension, as the 'locked back' knee position will affect the normal tibio-femoral angle, which in turn will affect the degree of lateral pelvic shift.[6] Excessive lateral shift is also usually associated with lack of hip extension which disturbs the normal body alignment at this point of stance phase and disrupts the mechanism which normally controls lateral shift.

3. **Inability to extend the affected hip** to shift the centre of gravity forward. When they first stand up, most patients have difficulty standing with their hips in the normal extended alignment. If hip extension is not trained specifically, the centre of gravity cannot be shifted forward normally when a step is taken with the **intact leg**, and two errors of movement occur in compensation. (a) Weight is not shifted forward until the intact foot is on the ground. (b) Weight is shifted forward not by extension of the affected leg but by extension of the intact leg with the affected hip in a flexed position. When a step is taken with the **affected leg**, another error occurs in compensation. Instead of weight being shifted forward on to the affected leg by extension at the hips, the patient flexes

his trunk forward on his affected hip and takes a short step forward with his intact leg.

Lack of hip extension, by affecting normal alignment, also makes impossible the control of the knee through the 0–15° necessary during stance phase, and causes the patient to shift his weight too far laterally. In some patients, extension of the hip may be prevented by excessive plantarflexor activity which prevents the centre of gravity from being shifted forward at a dorsiflexed ankle.

4. **Lack of knee control** throughout stance phase. When the patient first takes weight through his affected leg, the knee usually collapses into flexion because of a lack of control over the knee extensors in their inner range. He will soon learn to compensate by passively levering his knee into its fully extended position and keeping it there until the end of stance phase (see Fig. 8.6). This distorts the normally smooth progression of walking brought about by the 'yield' of the knee and prevents the patient from flexing his knee prior to the start of swing phase. The problem results from an inability to contract the quadriceps and control knee extension through 0–15°. It is augmented by inability to extend the hip and, once the patient has mastered this, he may find it easier to control his knee throughout stance. Some patients develop excessive plantarflexor activity and this will prevent hip extension and shift of the centre of gravity forward at the ankle, and the knee will be kept in a stiffly extended position. Occasionally, a patient may be seen to walk with his knee held in slight flexion during the stance phase. This is usually a learned response resulting from a failure to train knee control and substitution of one movement error for another.

Control over the knee during stance is very complex, requiring first an eccentric or lengthening contraction of the quadriceps, then a concentric contraction to extend the knee just prior to knee flexion. Knee control must therefore be trained specifically with this complex function in mind.

5. **Lack of knee flexion at toe-off** (see Fig. 8.8) is a major problem which, due to the patient's attempts at compensation, distorts the entire sequence of swing phase. Normally, knee flexion occurs at the end of stance phase while the hip is in an extended position. This action decreases the moment of inertia of the lower extremity. Inability to flex the knee at this point produces in compensation an abnormal swing forward of the affected leg, which involves hitching of the pelvis, abduction of the hip and backward tilting of the pelvis. In analysing this phase, it may appear that lack of hip flexion is the major problem. However, although the patient may indeed lack a few degrees of flexion at the hip, once he has gained sufficient active knee flexion to allow his foot to clear the ground, hip flexion will be seen to be quite sufficient for walking. Hip flexion may need to be trained later in rehabilitation in order that the patient can gain sufficient hip movement to step over objects and walk up stairs.

6. **Lack of dorsiflexion** should not be considered as a problem to be

treated in isolation. The major activity in the dorsiflexors normally occurs in stance phase just after heel strike and, although they are active before this, it is the flexion of the knee and hip which 'shortens' the leg and allows the foot to clear the ground at the start of swing phase. Hence, if the patient drags his foot during swing phase, the major missing component to be trained will be knee flexion. Lack of dorsiflexion on heel strike must be trained specifically in combination with the knee extension which normally accompanies it.

7. **A wide base** during practice of stepping forward or walking occurs principally due to poor balance and a fear of falling and will, therefore, be overcome by balance training with the feet closer together, that is, under the hips. However, in the early stages, it may also be due to the patient's inability to control the affected leg during swing phase (see Fig. 8.9). The compensatory movements which occur due to inability to flex the knee at toe-off may result in the affected foot being placed in a relatively abducted position. In addition, in stance phase, the poor alignment which results from lack of hip extension and excessive lateral horizontal shift towards the affected side may result in the intact foot stepping out to the side.

If the walking section of this Programme is to be effective, it is essential that the analysis of problems is accurate and that the correct decisions are made as to the most essential components to be trained (which should be those components upon which many other components depend), and the sequence in which they are trained. For example, the patient may lack rotation of his pelvis forward on the affected side during stance (i.e. external rotation of the weight-bearing hip). This, however, results from lack of hip extension and this is the component to be trained. Hip rotation normally occurs in conjunction with hip extension in stance and in monitoring the patient's alignment as he practises taking a step forward, the therapist will find an explanation to him about keeping the pelvis in line (i.e. by extending his hip), plus manual guidance, will be sufficient to ensure that the correct movement takes place. The use of resistance to walking in an attempt to promote rotation will distort the walking action by giving excessive emphasis to rotation. Walking against resistance is not indicated for stroke patients as it stimulates incorrect muscle activity and interferes with the complex learning process.

Loss of two or more components (determinants) makes effective compensation impossible.[1] Hence, it is important to recognise the most essential missing components, to concentrate on these in training and to discourage the patient from attempting to walk by himself while he is still unable to perform these components. If he does practise walking without these components, he will be unable to compensate effectively and will learn to walk abnormally and ineffectively. It is the authors' experience that most patients following stroke are capable of learning these components quickly if they are specifically trained in the early stages.

**STEP 2    PRACTICE OF MISSING COMPONENTS**

The reader should refer to the section on Balanced Standing (p. 102), as there is an overlap between these two sections.

**Stance Phase**

**To Stimulate Hip Extension**
See p. 106.

**To Train Knee Control**

*Sitting (supine if hamstrings are tight), with knee held at 0°, therapist gives firm pressure through heel towards knee while patient (i) practises controlling an eccentric and concentric contraction of the quadriceps through a 15° range (Fig. 8.11), and (ii) attempts to keep knee straight. Pressure through the heel must be as firm as possible in order to simulate weight-bearing, and to allow quadriceps to contract eccentrically on flexion.*

NOTE
It may be easier for the patient to activate his knee extensors (to keep his knee from bending further) with his knee held at 15° or 20° first, then to further straighten it a few degrees, bend it again, and so on until he is practising in the required 0° to 15° range.

INSTRUCTIONS
(i) 'Bend your knee a little—not too much. Now straighten it.'
(ii) 'Try to keep your knee straight.'

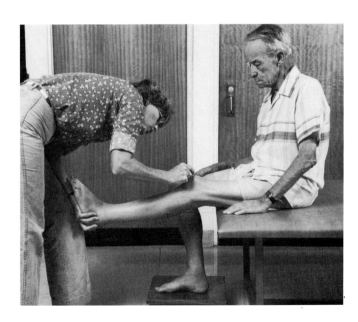

**Fig. 8.11** *Patient practises flexing and extending his knee through 0–15° to improve control over his quadriceps.*

CHECK

Make sure the patient's leg is positioned so that the bed does not block full knee extension and to allow hip as well as knee movement. It is the thigh that moves, not the lower leg.

Do not allow knee movement to become jerky or uncontrolled.

(i) The patient should practise the part of the range he can just control, increasing the controllable range as soon as possible.

(ii) As soon as he has some control at 0°, he practises holding his knee at varying positions between 0° and 15°.

In (ii) the knee must not be 'locked' into extension.

Do not allow him to plantarflex his foot.

Followed by:

*Patient stands up and practises stepping forward and backwards with intact leg.*

INSTRUCTIONS

'Keep your weight on this (affected) side.'

'Take a step forward.'

'Keep your knee straight. Now, step back.'

CHECK

Patient must stand up with weight on affected leg.

Make sure he keeps knee controlled throughout stepping.

Do not allow him to step out to the side. He must step directly forward.

Make sure hip remains extended throughout and moves forward as patient steps forward.

Stride should be of average length.

The following will add variety to practice and further train knee control.

*Patient places intact foot on 8 cm (3 in) step.*

INSTRUCTIONS

'Put your L/R foot on to the step.'

'Keep your hip straight.'

'Put your foot back down again.'

CHECK

Ensure that centre of gravity is not shifted backwards as patient flexes intact leg, i.e. affected hip must be extended throughout.

Do not allow affected knee to flex or hyperextend.

Do not allow him to step out to the side.

*Standing with affected foot on step. Patient shifts weight forward and steps up on to step and down again with intact leg (Fig. 8.12). Progress to stepping over.*

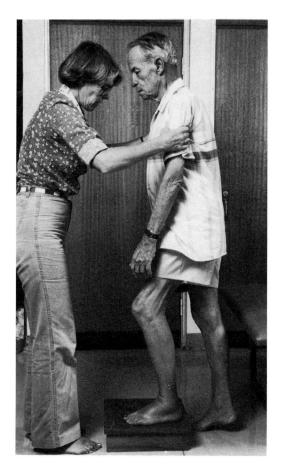

**Fig. 8.12** *This man, with the therapist's guidance, is shifting his centre of gravity forward over his affected foot before stepping up.*

INSTRUCTIONS
'Put this (affected) foot on to the step.'
'Bring your hips forward and step up.'
'Keep your knee bent until your weight is forward.'
'Now, straighten your knee.'

CHECK
Do not allow knee to extend prematurely, i.e. knee must not be extended until weight is far enough forward.
Make sure his affected leg does the movement and that he does not push up with intact leg.
Do not allow him to step out to the side.
When stepping over, he must not put his toes down first, and he must extend his affected knee fully before bending it to lower the foot to the ground.

NOTE
The above can also be used to train the movements required for walking on stairs.

*Standing with intact leg in front of affected leg (Fig. 8.13). Patient practises shifting his hips forward and backwards while maintaining knee extension of the affected leg. The step size should be small or it will be inappropriate to keep the knee extended. The patient may get a better idea of how to control his knee if he flexes his knee a few degrees then extends it. Weight must be forward over the intact leg as he practises this.*

INSTRUCTIONS
'Move your hips forward.'
'Keep your knee straight.'
'Practise bending and straightening your knee a few degrees. Keep your weight forward.'

CHECK
Make sure affected knee remains straight—as hips are moved forward it may tend to flex passively.

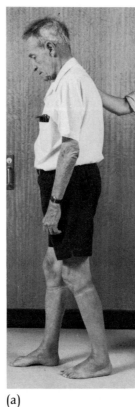 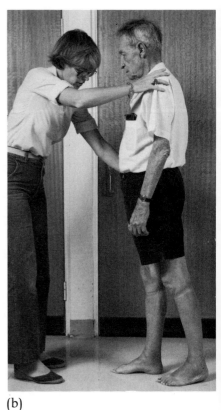

(a)                              (b)

**Fig. 8.13(a)** *This man's affected L. knee has flexed before his weight is sufficiently forward.* **(b)** *Therapist assists him to shift weight and reminds him to keep his L. knee straight.*

## To Train Lateral Horizontal Pelvic Shift

*In standing, hips over feet, patient practises shifting his weight from one side to the other in a small range (Fig. 8.14a). The therapist indicates with her finger how far he should move, i.e. 2½ cm (approximately 1 in).*

INSTRUCTIONS
'Shift your hips to this side—not too much. Now to the other side—just a little.'

CHECK
Make sure hips and knees remain extended.
Do not allow him to shift his weight too far to the side.

*In standing, hips over feet, patient practises stepping forward with intact leg (Fig. 8.14b) while therapist helps him control the amount of lateral pelvic shift.*

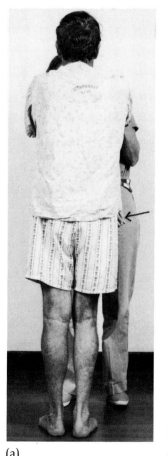 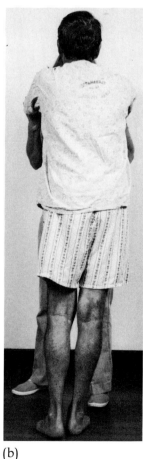

(a)                    (b)

**Fig. 8.14(a)** *This man is practising shifting his pelvis laterally to his affected R. side. Note the therapist's finger indicating the small range of movement required* **(b)** *Here, he is about to take a step forward with the L. leg. Note that at this point he needs to control not only the lateral pelvic shift but also his hip and knee extension. His excessive lateral shift is associated with flexion of the hip and hyperextension of the knee.*

Another way to stimulate controlled lateral weight shift is as follows.

*Walking sideways. For example, therapist with one hand at patient's L. waist helps him to shift his weight towards the R. He takes a step sideways to the L. (Fig. 8.15). As he does, the therapist, with one hand at his waist, helps him shift his weight towards the L. over the L. leg. Patient adducts his R. leg to take its place next to the L.*

NOTE

If the patient cannot abduct his affected leg to step, therapist helps him, using her own foot to guide the movement once weight is shifted to the support leg. If necessary, patient can rest his arms on the therapist's shoulders. This gives him a little support. His elbows should be extended and he should not hang on around the therapist's neck.

INSTRUCTIONS

'Let's walk sideways. Weight over to the R. and step sideways with your L. foot. Shift your hips to the L.—not too far. Now, feet together.'

CHECK

Make sure shoulders remain level and over the hips.
Hips must remain extended—he must progress sideways not diagonally.
He must not shift his pelvis too far laterally.

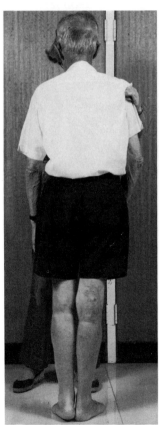
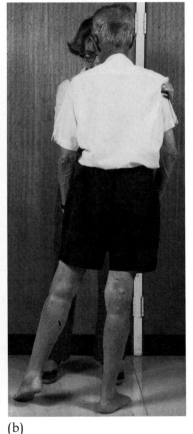

**Fig. 8.15(a) and (b)** *This man is taking a step to the L. The therapist's hands, at his waist and shoulders, guide the movement and indicate the alignment necessary. As he shifts his weight to the L. leg, the therapist will change her hands to the opposite shoulder and waist. Note that this man has not yet gained the ability to shift his weight to the L. simultaneously with the L. hip abduction.*

(a)                    (b)

## Swing Phase

### To Train Flexion of Knee at Start of Swing Phase

*Prone on bed, therapist flexes knee to just below a right angle. Patient practises controlling his knee flexors both eccentrically and concentrically throughout a small range of movement (Fig. 8.16).*

NOTE

With the knee at a right angle, it is usually easier for the patient to contract the knee flexors. As the patient gains control around this point, he is encouraged to increase the range of movement. He must try actively to gain control over his hamstrings throughout their middle range. Firm pounding to the heel may make the patient more aware of where his leg is in space. The therapist must ensure that the hip does not flex as the patient attempts to activate his knee flexors. The patient may only be able to activate them in conjunction with hip flexion and not under any other circumstance, and this is not compatible with normal function. The therapist should keep in mind the effect a tight rectus femoris muscle will have on the range of knee flexion which is possible without the hip flexing.

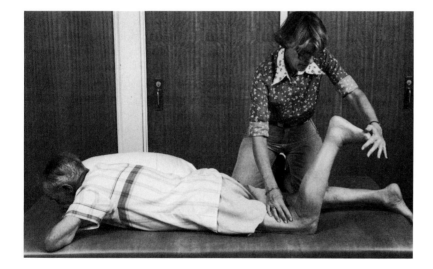

**Fig. 8.16** *Patient practises controlling knee flexors.*

INSTRUCTIONS

'Try to hold your knee there—bend it up a little—now let it down slowly. Bend it up again. Don't be jerky—make a smooth slow movement. Don't move your hip.'

CHECK

Do not allow jerky uncontrolled movement. Therapist assists by taking some of the weight of the leg.
Do not allow the hip to flex.

Followed by:

*Standing, therapist holds patient's knee in some flexion. He practises controlled eccentric and concentric knee flexion (Fig. 8.17).*

NOTE

It is often easier for the patient to take his toes down to the floor (an eccentric contraction of his knee flexors) **before** lifting them up from the floor (a concentric contraction).

**Fig. 8.17** *Patient practises controlling knee flexion in preparation for stepping forward.*

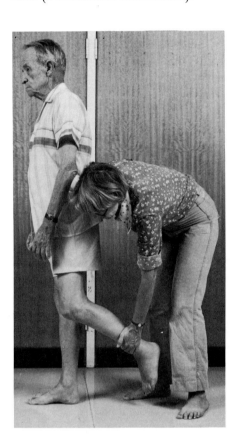

INSTRUCTIONS

'Give me your leg. Don't let your hip bend.'
'Let your toes go down to touch the floor—gently—do it again, just a short distance. Now bend your knee again. Lift your toes up off the floor.'

CHECK

Do not flex his knee too much. This will pull him off balance, and tension on his rectus femoris will cause his hip to flex as well as making it difficult for him to contract his knee flexors.

Do not allow hip to bend more than a few degrees.

Do not push the patient off balance—hold his opposite arm, and make sure his weight is over his standing foot.

Followed by:

*Patient steps forward with affected leg, therapist helping him control the initial knee flexion.*

INSTRUCTIONS
'Bend your knee.'
'Step forward. Heel down first.'

CHECK
Make sure the patient shifts weight forward as he takes a step.

*Patient walks backwards. Therapist guides knee flexion and foot dorsiflexion (Fig. 8.18).*

INSTRUCTIONS
'Bend your knee, take your leg back and put your toes to the ground.'
'Walk backwards.'

CHECK
Do not allow patient to incline trunk forward at hips.
He should step backwards one leg after the other in a rhythmical manner.

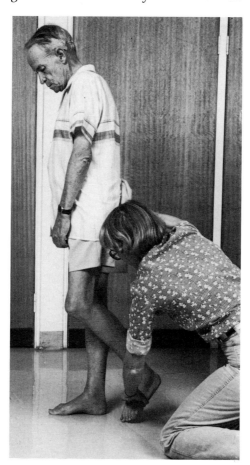

**Fig. 8.18** *Practice of walking backward. Therapist uses R. hand to ensure hip extension. She guides knee flexion and foot dorsiflexion of L. leg.*

### To Stimulate Knee Extension and Foot Dorsiflexion at Heel Strike

*Patient standing on intact leg, therapist holds the patient's affected foot in dorsiflexion, with the knee in extension, and shifts his weight forward to stimulate stepping forward with heel down first (Fig. 8.19).*

NOTE

This technique frequently elicits tibialis anterior and toe extensor activity even when this cannot be elicited in any other way.

INSTRUCTIONS

'Let me have your foot. Don't hold yourself stiffly, I won't let you fall. I'm going to shift your weight forward so you step forward on to your heel.'

CHECK

Do not allow the patient to pull back when you are trying to shift his weight forward.

Do not allow him to bend the other knee. He will do this if the therapist does not shift his weight or if he pulls back.

Ensure that step length is not too long.

Do not give too many instructions. You are trying to elicit an automatic response.

NOTE

This technique can also be used, with the intact foot forward, to train control of knee extension of the affected leg during stance phase.

**Fig. 8.19(a)** *Therapist guides weight shift forward while holding the affected foot in dorsiflexion.* **(b)** *At heel strike, the alignment of both lower limbs is incorrect. Weight is too far back and his R. knee is flexed.* **(c)** *Training consists of instructing patient to keep his R. knee straight and to allow his weight to be shifted forward. Now when he is moved forward he is able to maintain improved alignment.*

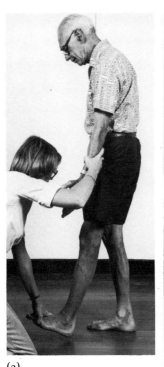
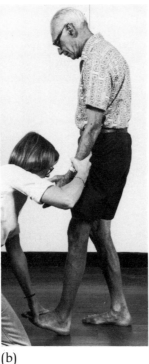
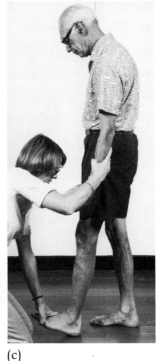

(a)                    (b)                    (c)

### STEP 3   PRACTICE OF WALKING

Practice of individual components of walking should be followed by walking facilitation which enables the patient to put these components together in their proper sequence.

## Walking Facilitation*

*Therapist shifts patient's weight to the affected side and forward, at the same time rotating his body so the shoulder on the weight-bearing side is in front of the other. Weight shift forward is accomplished most effectively when the body is shifted forward as a whole from the ankles. This ensures that, as he steps forward, he does so with his body segments maintaining the correct alignment. As the heel touches the ground at the end of the swing phase, the therapist reverses the procedure.*

NOTE
It may be difficult for the patient to step forward with his affected leg, and the therapist, for the first few times, may need to guide his leg forward with her own. However, it is better if the procedure can be done rhythmically without other interference. This stimulation of the rhythm of walking may itself trigger off the missing components. Counting or saying 'right–left' or 'step–step' will help him to get the timing of the movement (Fig. 8.20). The patient should walk at an average speed. Walking slowly requires more control.

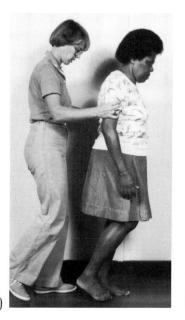 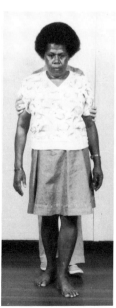

(a)                                                    (b)

**Fig. 8.20(a)** *The patient's weight is to the L. Therapist is shifting weight forward while rotating the upper trunk towards the right.* **(b)** *Note the position of therapist's hands and the patient's small base of support.*

*Based on a technique described by B. Bobath (1967) in *Techniques of Stimulating and Facilitating Spontaneous Movements*. Handout from the then Western Cerebral Palsy Centre, London.

INSTRUCTIONS
'I'm going to guide you as you walk so you can get the feeling of the rhythm of walking. Don't worry if you can't do it very well to begin with—the important thing is to **feel** how to walk.'

CHECK
Do not push the patient off balance.
Do not rotate the shoulders in the wrong direction.
Do not incline the trunk forward at the hips. Therapist must ensure normal body segment alignment throughout.
Do not shift weight too far laterally or the patient will abduct the non weight-bearing leg instead of stepping forward.
Do not get out of step yourself. When the patient steps forward with his R. leg, the therapist does the same.
Do not hold on to the patient too much.

## To Increase Complexity

The patient needs the opportunity to improve his walking skills. His new abilities must be constantly stretched to their limits, with the frequent addition to his programme of more complex activities. Below are some examples.

*Quick stepping in all directions. Patient rests his hands at the therapist's waist. The therapist, holding the patient's elbows straight, stimulates automatic stepping with quick, unpredictable changes in direction.*

*As above, but the therapist holds only the affected arm and stands further from the patient.*

*Patient practises stepping over objects of different heights. This can be done with manual guidance (as in walking facilitation) or with verbal feedback only. It is also a useful way of training hip flexion for walking up stairs and kerbs.*

*Walking combined with other activities such as conversation, carrying objects.*

*Varying the speed of walking and the spatial confines within which the person walks.*

*Treadmill walking is another way of improving the rhythm and timing of walking. It is also a useful method of increasing cardiopulmonary efficiency and endurance and of measuring these as a guide to progress. The treadmill should be adjusted to the most comfortable speed for each person.*

**STEP 4**     TRANSFERENCE OF LEARNING INTO DAILY LIFE

At the end of the therapy session, the therapist allows some time for the patient to walk at least part of the way to his next appointment by walking facilitation, if necessary, and as soon as possible he should walk alone.

The patient needs the opportunity to practise correctly with other members of staff and relatives what he has been learning in therapy and he will benefit from videotaped instructions between therapy sessions. Figure 8.21 illustrates one way of assisting the patient to walk. The therapist must ensure that staff do not interfere with the training process by giving the patient a four-point stick, by helping him from his intact side or by walking arm in arm.

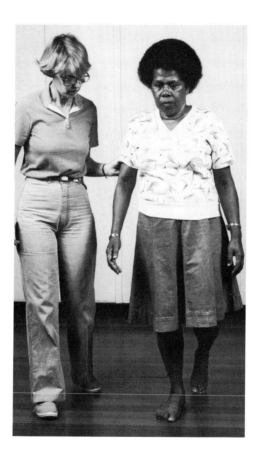

**Fig. 8.21** *This woman needs only a little guidance and verbal feedback. Note therapist's hand on upper arm. Slight elevation of the shoulder encourages weight shift with normal alignment.*

## REFERENCES

1. Saunders J. B., Inman V. T. and Eberhart H. D. (1953). The major determinants in normal and pathological gait. *J. Bone Jt Surg*; **35A,3**:543–58.
2. Dubo H. I. C., Peat M., Winter D. A., Quanbury A. O., Hobson D. A., Steinke T. and Reimer G. (1976). Electromyographic temporal analysis of gait: normal human locomotion. *Arch. phys. Med;* **57**:415–20.
3. Winter D. A. (1979). *Biomechanics of Human Movement*. New York: John Wiley.
4. Milner M., Basmajian J. V. and Quanbury A. O. (1971). Multifactorial analysis of walking by electromyography and computer. *Amer. J. phys. Med*; **50**:235–58.
5. Battye C. K. and Joseph J. (1966). An investigation by telemetering of the activity of some muscles in walking. *Med biol. Engng*; **4**:125–35.
6. Eberhard H. D., Inman V. T. and Bresler B. (1969). The principal elements in human locomotion. In *Human Limbs and their Substitutes* (Klopstag P. F. and Wilson D. P., eds.) pp. 437–471. New York: McGraw Hill.
7. Herman R., Cook T., Cozzens B. and Freedman W. (1973). Control of postural reactions in man: the initiation of gait. In *Control of Posture and Locomotion* (Stein R. B. *et al.*, eds.) pp. 363–388. New York: Plenum Press.
8. Pearson K. (1976) The control of walking. *Scientific American;* **December**:72–86.
9. Murray M. P., Drought A. B. and Kory R. C. (1964). Walking patterns of normal men. *J. Bone Jt Surg*; **46A,2**:335–60.
10. Kramer J. F. and Reid D. C. (1981). Backward walking: a cinematographic and electromyographic pilot study. *Physiotherapy Canada*; **33,2**:77–86.
11. Andriacchi T. P., Andersson G. B. J., Fermier R. W., Stern D. and Galante J. O. (1980). A study of lower limb mechanics during stair-climbing. *J. Bone Jt Surg*; **62A**:749–57.

## FURTHER READING

Aptekar R. G., Ford F. and Bleck E. E. (1976). Light patterns as a means of assessing and recording gait: methods and results in normal children. *Develop. Med. Child Neurol*; **18**:31–6.

Carlsöö S. (1966). The initiation of walking. *Acta anat*; **65**:1–9.

Holt K. S., Jones R. B. and Wilson R. (1974). Gait analysis by means of a multiple sequential exposure camera. *Develop. Med. Child Neurol*; **16**:742–5.

Inman V. T. (1947). Functional aspects of the abductor muscles of the hip. *J. Bone Jt Surg*; **29**:607–19.

Murray M. P., Drought A. B. and Kory R. C. (1969). Walking patterns in healthy old men. *J. Geront*; **24**:169–78.

Robinson J. L. and Smidt G. L. (1981). Quantitative gait evaluation in the clinic. *Arch. phys. Med*; **61**:351–3.

Van Ingen Schenau G. J. (1980). Some fundamental aspects of the biomechanics of overground versus treadmill locomotion. *Medicine and Science in Sports and Exercise*; **12**:257–61.

Winter D. A. (1981). Use of kinetic analysis in the diagnostics of pathological gait. *Physiotherapy Canada*; **3**:209–30.

# PART III

# Appendices

# Appendix 1

# Mechanisms of recovery

Although little is actually known of what occurs in the brain following damage to its structure, it is probable that recovery can occur as a result of changes in neural organisation which take place in response to injury. A number of hypothetical considerations of adaptation and reorganisation are to be found in the literature.[1-11] Anatomical evidence supports the notion that new central connections are formed.[12-14] Certainly, the often impressive degree of recovery of function seen in adults following even apparently extensive lesions of the brain suggests that changes are occurring within the nervous system.

Some of the theories and mechanisms which have been proposed to account for recovery following brain damage are as follows.

1. **von Monakow's diaschisis theory.** This is a theory of a temporary traumatic disruption of neural organisation and integration, which is a type of 'functional shock'.[15] This theory suggests that the widespread effects of such processes as oedema and extracellular blood flow cause a suppression of activity in areas far from the site of the lesion. Similarly, reversible changes may occur in undamaged synapses resulting in a temporary impairment of neural transmission. This theory could account for any recovery of function in the early period following a lesion.

2. Another theory which may provide part of the explanation for early recovery is that of **denervation supersensitivity**. The axons and terminals degenerate following a lesion and the denervated part of the target cells may develop an increased post-synaptic responsiveness to neurotransmitter substances, becoming increasingly sensitive to the remaining afferent input.[9]

3. **Redundancy theory.**[16] Several parts of the central nervous system may mediate the same motor function. That is, a part of a neural system may adequately mediate the function normally subserved by the system as a whole. Lashley[17] had a similar concept which he called equipotentiality. He suggested that a particular function was mediated by all the tissues in a given region. If part of that region was damaged, the remaining intact tissue would continue to mediate that function. The effect of the

lesion would therefore depend more on the **amount** of tissue spared than on the **location** of the lesion.

4. **Vicarious function.** The intact system may have had a latent capacity to control the functions which are lost. After a lesion these latent functions would become overt.[9]

5. **Functional reorganisation.** It is possible that a neural system can change its functions qualitatively, in which case a neural pathway could take over the control of some motor behaviour not ordinarily part of its repertoire.[9]

6. Two forms of **neural sprouting** within the central nervous system have been suggested. (a) **Regeneration**, which refers to new growth in damaged neurons. The newly generated axons may re-innervate the denervated areas. (b) **Collateral sprouting**, in which there is new growth in undamaged neurons adjacent to destroyed neural tissue. Sprouting would increase synaptic effectiveness and allow the new system to substitute for the destroyed synapses. The emergence of new synaptic connections may be indicative of a dynamic synaptogenesis which is continually occurring under normal circumstances,[12] enabling the organism to adjust in the face of continually changing environmental needs. These widespread synaptic changes may be the underlying physiological mechanism for a relearning or compensatory process which is actually responsible for recovery and is no more fundamental than the changes which occur in any learning situation.[18] Laurence and Stein[15] suggest that it is possible that in the normal brain 'cells may die leaving a number of vacated sites which can be filled by intact cells. In this way, the mature brain may differ from the immature one by virtue of the greater number and complexity of its interneural connections and elaboration made at the expense of absolute cell numbers'.[15]

7. **Behavioural strategy change.** This is a form of **substitution**, in which the strategy utilised in order to achieve a motor goal is different. Other forms of substitution may involve the use of a different sensory cue for guiding movement, or a functional substitution in which the recovered movements are produced differently from the lost movements, although they are essentially the same.[19] Certainly, one of the problems in research in this area is the difficulty in identifying whether recovery is due to anatomical and physiological changes or to the use of alternative or compensatory strategies by the subject.

Other theories suggest that previously ineffective synapses may become effective following disruption of input to nerve cells, and that there may be spontaneous changes in inhibitory activity. This process may explain in part the recovery from the stage of depressed motor activity or 'cerebral shock'. Chemical changes may occur which enhance the process of synaptic modification.[10] Studies being carried out by Goldberger[9] indicate that motor recovery after a lesion may not be a diffuse process but a process which is regulated hierarchically.

Assuming that the brain is capable of adaptation and reorganisation, what happens to the patient following stroke must be exceedingly important. Luria[19] suggests that an essential condition of such re-organisation is that a particular activity practised be necessary and he states that the greater the need, the more automatically and easily will reorganisation be carried out. Singer[20] comments that '. . . if certain patterns of movement have been established before injury or disease occurs, there is a better chance neurons in surrounding areas will be able to compensate for their loss of function'. Just as it can be assumed that early practice of relevant motor skills takes advantage of the brain's plasticity, so it is also possible that lack of relevant practice can allow secondary neuronal atrophy to occur.[4,14]

Whether or not the MRP stimulates anatomical and physiological reorganisation or whether it enables the patient to take advantage of it is, of course, open to question. The authors' clinical experience suggests that patients on this specific programme of motor learning, which should commence within the first few days following stroke, make a more impressive recovery of function with less reflex hyperactivity than patients receiving more 'traditional' physiotherapy. This may be due to the emphasis both on very early training of specific control of those muscles of the affected limbs which are essential for function and which tend to be disadvantaged, as well as on elimination of overuse of the intact side and of unnecessary muscle activity of the affected side.

Two other factors which may exert a profound influence upon recovery and which need investigation are the effect on recovery of the quality of the brain before the lesion occurred, and of the quality of the environment in which the patient finds himself following his lesion.[21-24]

### REFERENCES

1. Raisman G. (1969). Neuronal plasticity in the septal nuclei of the adult rat. *Brain Res*; **14**:15–48
2. Wall P. D. and Egger M. D. (1971). Formation of new connexions in the adult rat brains after partial deafferentation. *Nature*; **232**:542–545.
3. Brodal A. (1973). Self-observations and neuro-anatomical considerations after a stroke. *Brain*; **96** (Part IV):675–694.
4. Eccles J. C. (1973). *The Understanding of the Brain*. New York: McGraw Hill.
5. Stein D. G., Rosen J. J. and Butters N., eds. (1974). *Plasticity and Recovery of Function in the Central Nervous System*. New York: Academic Press.
6. Goldman P. S. (1974). An alternative to developmental plasticity: heterology of CNS structures in infants and adults. In *Plasticity and Recovery of Function in the Central Nervous System* (Stein D. G., Rosen J. J. and Butters N., eds.) pp. 149–174. New York: Academic Press.
7. Finger S. (1978). *Recovery from Brain Damage*. London: Plenum Press.
8. Székely G. (1979). Order and plasticity in the nervous system. *Trends in Neuroscience*; **2**:245–8.
9. Goldberger M. (1980). Motor recovery after lesions. *Trends in Neuroscience*; **3**:288–91.

10. Kasamatsu T., Pettigrew J. D. and Ary M. (1981). Cortical recovery from effects of monocular deprivation: acceleration with Norepinephrine and suppression with 6-Hydroxydopamine. *J. Physiol*; **45**:1.

11. Miles F. A. and Lisberger S. G. (1981). Plasticity in the vestibulo-ocular reflex: a new hypothesis. *Ann. Rev. Neurosc*; **4**:273–299.

12. Chambers W. W., Liu C. N. and McCouch G. P. (1973). Anatomical and physiological correlates of plasticity in the central nervous system. *Brain, Behaviour and Evolutions*; **8**:5–26.

13. Kerr F. W. L. (1975). Structural and functional evidence for plasticity in the central nervous system. *Exp. Neur*; **48**:16–31.

14. Woolsey T. A. (1978). Lesion experiments: some anatomical considerations. In *Recovery from Brain Damage* (Finger S., ed.) pp. 71–89. London: Plenum Press.

15. Laurence S. and Stein D. G. (1978). Recovery after brain damage and the concept of localisation of function. In *Recovery from Brain Damage* (Finger S., ed.) pp. 369–407. London: Plenum Press.

16. Rosner B. S. (1970). Brain functions. *Ann. Rev. Psych*; **21**:555–594.

17. Lashley K. S. (1979). *Brain Mechanisms and Intelligence*. Chicago: University of Chicago Press.

18. Bliss T. V. P. (1979). Synaptic plasticity in the hippocampus. *Trends in Neuroscience*; **2**:42–45.

19. Luria A. R. (1963). *Restoration of Function after Brain Injury*. London: Pergamon.

20. Singer R. N. (1980). *Motor Learning and Human Performance*, 3rd edn. New York: Macmillan.

21. Rosenzweig M. R., Bennett E. L. and Diamond M. C. (1967). Effects of differential environments on brain anatomy and brain chemistry. *Proc. Amer. psychopath. Ass*; **56**:45–6.

22. Goldman P. S. (1976). The role of experience in recovery of function following orbital prefrontal lesion in infant monkeys. *Neuropsychologia*; **14**:401–12.

23. Rosenzweig M. R. and Bennett E. L. (1978). Experimental influences on brain anatomy and brain chemistry in rodents. In *Studies on the Development of Behaviour and the Nervous System* (Gottlieb G., ed.) pp. 289–327. New York: Academic Press.

24. Walsh R. (1981). Sensory environments, brain damage, and drugs: a review of the interactions and mediating mechanisms. *Int. J. Neuroscience*; **14**:129–37.

# Appendix 2

# Elimination of unnecessary muscle activity

In the very early stages following stroke, the patient demonstrates an inability to move, that is, to activate muscles, on the affected side. This depression of motor function[1] is referred to as transient flaccidity or hypotonia, although sometimes the misleading terms of paralysis or weakness are used.

Gradually there is a return of muscular activity. From the moment activity can first be elicited, there is a tendency for the patient to make four types of error in using the recovering muscles and these errors are augmented by the effort he uses as he tries hard to accomplish the desired activity.

1. He may tend to activate the wrong muscle for a particular activity.

2. He may make too strong a contraction for the needs of the movement.

3. He may move the intact side instead of the affected side.

4. He may demonstrate a spread of synergic muscle/activity* in fairly predictable patterns (associated movements reactions[2]).

His attempts to move have, therefore, the opposite to the desired effect, making the required activity even harder to accomplish.

The authors' clinical experience with stroke patients suggests that the degree of stereotyped and excessive motor activity demonstrated by a patient and the amount of motor control he is able to regain may depend as much on his experience following the stroke as upon the actual brain damage—that is, the pathophysiological effects of the stroke itself.[3,4] These experiences include the patient's own attempts to move, the way in which he is assisted to move by relatives and staff, his environment and the type of physiotherapy he receives.

---

*The synergies seen in a stroke patient seem to have a positional component. For example, a person who is left in the sitting position tends to develop flexor overactivity in the lower limb; a person who stands early without bearing weight through the affected leg tends to develop extensor overactivity in this leg. The muscles which tend to become overactive seem to be the muscles which, in terms of limb position, have the greatest advantage. Hence, the development of muscle imbalance may, to some extent, be dependent upon certain muscles being in a better 'postion' to recover function, with certain other muscles (their antagonists) tending *not* to recover function because of their relative disadvantage.

It is probable that these experiences, occurring in conjunction with reorganisation of the brain, affect recovery, either positively, by actually stimulating reorganisation itself or by enabling the patient to take advantage of it, or negatively, by retarding or interfering with reorganisation. That is, the patient's experiences, if they are positive, will trigger off a learning process which may itself be an important factor in the brain's reorganisation. However, whether he learns to move correctly or incorrectly will depend on the training he receives. Practice of inappropriate muscle activity will result in the wrong movement being trained, and in a sense so-called 'spasticity' is made up of habitual, incorrect and unnecessary motor responses.

The re-emergence of motor activity in individual muscles is therefore a crucial event in terms of the patient's eventual recovery of function. At this time, the physiotherapist should be stimulating the recovery of the muscle activity necessary for specific functions and ensuring that there is not an unbalanced recovery of activity in certain muscles which do not normally function together. The direction which recovery of muscle activity following stroke takes—that is, into abnormal synergies or into normal functional movements—probably depends to a large extent upon physiotherapy at this stage.

Many authors[5-7] stress the importance of motor learning consisting as much of inhibition of unnecessary activity as of activation of more units. Broer and Zernicke[8] comment that muscular control involves the ability to relax, i.e. the ability to prevent muscles which do not contribute to the maintenance of the position or the execution of the movement from contracting. They suggest that the ability to relax is as much a motor skill as any movement. Blomfield and Marr[9] suggest that movements are learned by the turning off of incorrect elemental movements, and MacConaill and Basmajian[10] that expenditure of energy should be the minimum necessary to allow the desired activity to be achieved.

Kottke and co-workers[11] comment that motor patterns 'involve inhibition of neuronal pathways which should not be participating in the pattern, as well as excitation of the internuncial neurons leading to all the anterior horn cells needed in the pattern', and they go on to say that inhibition of undesired activity is more difficult than initiation of the desired activity. 'Trained inhibition', as they call it, prevents overflow of activity to other motor units and they caution that effort 'must be kept low during learning to avoid irradiation of excitation across the CNS'. The antagonist normally relaxes during a trained movement.[12] Failure to do so indicates lack of skill but it also indicates lack of motor control in the brain-damaged person.

Taub and Berman[13] point out that rehabilitation therapy could be described as additive in nature, depending on the belief that recovery of function can be achieved solely through the re-education or exercise of inactivated muscle groups. Their research with animals suggests that at least some motor deficits are caused 'not by the loss of nervous tissue as such, but rather by the unrestrained hyperactivity of certain neural centres, resulting in a disabling imbalance'.

Bobath,[2, 14] with her development of the techniques called 'reflex inhibiting movements', was a pioneer in the physiotherapy literature in emphasising the need to decrease 'tone' by 'inhibiting abnormal patterns of movement'.

## Overflow

In the intact person, an overflow of activity into muscles not necessary for the task is an indication of lack of motor skill. Overflow is seen in the normal child as an indication of his motor immaturity and in the normal adult who is learning a novel motor task. Overflow is called by various terms in the literature, including synkinetic movements, associated movements and associated reactions.[2,15–17] In the brain-damaged person, however, this irradiation of muscle activity on the affected side occurs principally in certain muscle groups. It augments the tendency towards excessive and inappropriate motor activity and imposes upon the patient the necessity for movement to be stereotyped, certain muscles always contracting in conjunction with certain other muscles.

In the early stages following stroke, this abnormal motor activity may be obvious as the patient attempts to move. For example, when he attempts to grasp an object, the initial extension, which is necessary to position the fingers correctly, may be absent. The fingers may flex before the object is in the hand, and there will also be an overflow of muscular activity into the wrist flexors, thumb adductors and forearm pronators. These events make effective hand use impossible. It is important at this stage that both the therapist and the patient understand what is happening. They may both be delighted at the sight of some recovery of movement, and the patient may want to practise this abnormal activity. The therapist must explain to him that uncontrolled and generalised flexor activity will actually **prevent** him from regaining effective use of his hand, and she should work with him to establish control over the particular muscles needed for certain activities. Emphasis will be on certain important movement components (extension and radial deviation of the wrist, extension of the carpo-metacarpal joints with fingers slightly flexed, thumb abduction, forearm supination) and on helping the patient to prevent his every attempt at movement from being directed solely into his flexors, ulnar deviators and pronators.

Although overflow of muscle activity tends to occur in certain synergic muscle groups on the affected side, the patient may also demonstrate unnecessary muscle activity on the intact side. He may clench his fist, replicate the attempted movement, or stiffen his arm and leg, and this muscle activity must also be prevented if the patient is to develop motor control on his affected side.

It is probable that many therapeutic techniques in current use encourage the development of recovering muscle activity into stereotyped synergies and actually prevent the patient from re-establishing the best possible motor control. Below are some illustrations of this theory.

### 1. Stimulation of Mass Movement Patterns

The Jacksonian theory that movement not muscles is represented in the motor cortex, which is no longer held to be correct,[12,18,19] has probably been responsible for the emphasis in the past 30 years being on the stimulation of 'movements' and away from the stimulation of discrete muscles.

The suggestion that it is necessary to stimulate mass movements implies that human movement can be classified into relatively few 'patterns' of activity, when in reality movement is infinitely complex and variable. For example, the patterns of movement described by Knott and Voss[20] may take into account the anatomical arrangements of muscles but the movements are stereotyped and bear little resemblance to the complexities of normal function.

Many therapists fail to realise the need to stimulate muscle activity appropriately, that is, taking into account such details as the range of movement, leverage, the effect of gravity and the fact that each muscle has several component parts which are recruited in different functions at different times.[21] The patient may practise, and therefore learn, incorrect muscle use. For example, in lying, when he takes his arm from his side to above his head, muscle activity changes in response to the arm's changing relationship to gravity. In performing this activity normally, muscle work changes from concentric in one group to eccentric in the opposite group, and the ability to make this shift is essential for control and function. However, resistance to this movement will encourage the use of one group of muscles concentrically throughout the entire range of movement. Similarly, if a person lying with his arm flexed at 90° to his body takes his hand to touch his face, the triceps brachii will normally need to contract eccentrically, i.e. to lengthen. If the therapist gives resistance to the patient's attempts at touching his head, she is encouraging him, as in the former example, to learn incorrect motor function. She is also reinforcing the tendency to develop overactivity in the flexors of the upper limb.

Stimulation of mass movements has been suggested as a means of eliciting or facilitating a motor response, with the intention that these movements can then be refined as the patient regains motor function.[16] The problem is, however, that if a highly diffuse muscular pattern is used in this way, it is *this* pattern which will become learned. The diffuse pattern will then have to be eliminated by practice later on. It is preferable for the patient to receive more specific stimulation, i.e. to be trained to contract specific muscles as practice towards the learning of a particular functional activity.

### 2. Resisted Exercise

There is no evidence that activation of increasing numbers of motor units produces any improvement in motor control in the brain-damaged person. Norton and Sahrmann[22] postulate that use of these resistive techniques may decrease the ability of the patient both to activate muscles selectively and to cease muscle activity once initiated. They also suggest that unnecessary voluntary effort, at various stages during walking for example, may be a major contribution to walking dysfunction.

Since certain muscles demonstrate activity more obviously than other muscles in the early stage following stroke, resisted exercises tend to be directed towards these muscles. Hence, the potentially 'spastic' or overactive muscles become trained to the exclusion of their antagonists, resulting in the disabling muscular imbalance so typical following stroke.

### 3. Encouragement of Movement of the Intact Side to Assist the Affected Side

When the therapist encourages the patient to move his affected leg by using his intact leg or to pivot on his intact leg when standing up, manoeuvres which the patient is frequently taught in the belief that they will enable him to achieve some level of independence, she is in fact encouraging responses which will have a negative effect upon his potential recovery of independence. In being trained to replace use of his affected limb with use of his intact limb, he is learning *not* to use the affected limb ('learned non-use').[23] It is possible that this emphasis on the intact side will cause interhemispheric interference, resulting in an 'extinction' of motor function of the affected side. Furthermore, use of the intact limbs, particularly when associated with effort, results in muscle activity in the affected limbs, but only in certain synergies. Hence, these manoeuvres will encourage a disabling muscle imbalance.

### PREVENTION OF MUSCLE IMBALANCE

To use the MRP in such a way as to enable the patient to recover effective function without disabling muscle imbalance, the therapist must appreciate the need to notice and eliminate all muscle activity which is unnecessary to the movement or function being relearned. This includes the recognition and prevention of stereotyped and abnormal synergic activity even when it is relatively minimal and not grossly evident.

From the earliest stages of rehabilitation, the physiotherapist must ensure that motor activity is appropriate, and this requires a thorough understanding of normal muscle function. When the patient contracts incorrect muscles, he should receive immediate verbal feedback from the therapist who points out his error. The patient needs to understand that it is by relaxing muscles not required in the movement that he will learn how to activate the correct ones. Therefore, the therapist will point out to him not only where muscular activity is incorrect, but also when it is unnecessary. It is in this way that the therapist prevents muscle imbalance from developing, prevents 'learned non-use' of the affected limbs through overuse of the intact limbs, and enables the patient to regain motor control.

It is important not to confuse elimination of unnecessary activity with a generalised relaxation. It seems important in learning a task (that is, in the cognitive phase of learning a motor skill) that the person is mentally and physically 'ready' for action. Sometimes, some preparatory muscular activity is necessary to set the scene, so that the nervous system is not having to make a shift from an inactive to an active state. In pointing out unnecessary muscular activity to a patient who is practising a particular function, the therapist should not encourage a general relaxation but relaxation only of a particular muscle or muscle group which is interfering with effective performance of the function.

Weight-bearing through the affected leg in standing seems to have an inhibiting effect upon the development of extensor overactivity[2] but only if the limb and trunk are in normal alignment. Anderson and Kottke[24] suggest that standing stimulates the internuncial pool, thus stimulating the appropriate motor function. Standing in correct alignment (that is, with the line of gravity falling in front of the ankle joints) also preserves length in the calf muscles, which may be another factor in the inhibition of extensor overactivity. The MRP emphasises the need to practise stepping forward with the intact leg while weight-bearing through the affected leg, particularly during the first therapy sessions. This seems to train the correct muscular response throughout the limb, which therefore would inhibit the tendency towards combined contraction of extensor and plantarflexor muscles.

The Programme also emphasises weight-bearing through the arm, particularly with the limb in the horizontal plane. This preserves length in the finger, wrist and elbow flexors, which develop contractures very quickly if flexor overactivity is not controlled, since the resting posture of the upper limb favours flexor activity. Once the patient has regained some active control over his wrist and finger extensors, weight-bearing is no longer necessary except as part of training for particular functions. The four-point kneeling position[25] is not recommended for adult patients as a position in which to gain weight-bearing. It is an unnecessarily complicated and difficult position for stimulating weight-bearing through the arms when this can be done so easily in functionally more appropriate positions such as sitting and standing.

## REFERENCES

1. Denny-Brown D. and Botterell E. H. (1948). The motor functions of the agranular frontal cortex. *A. Res. Nerv. & Ment. Dis. Proc*; **27**:235.
2. Bobath B. (1959). Observations on adult hemiplegia and suggestions for treatment. *Physiotherapy*; **45**:279–89.
3. Carr J. H. and Shepherd R. B. (1980). *Physiotherapy in Disorders of the Brain*. London: Heinemann Medical.
4. Shepherd R. (1979). Some factors influencing the outcome of stroke rehabilitation. *Aust. J. Physiother*; **25**:4.
5. Basmajian J. V. (1976). Electromyographic investigation of spasticity and muscle spasm. *Physiotherapy*; **62**:319–23.
6. O'Connell A. L. (1972). *Understanding the Scientific Basis for Human Movement*. Baltimore: Williams and Wilkins.
7. Bruner J. S. (1973). Organisation of early skilled action. *Child Develop*; **44**(4):1–11.

8.  Broer M. R. and Zernicke R. F. (1979) *Efficiency of Human Movement*, 4th edn. Philadelphia: W. B. Saunders.

9.  Blomfield S. and Marr D. (1970). How the cerebellum may be used. *Nature*; **227**:1224–8.

10. MacConaill M. A. and Basmajian J. V. (1969). *Muscles and Movements. Basis for Human Kinesiology*. Baltimore: Williams and Wilkins.

11. Kottke F. J., Halpern D., Easton, J., Ozel A. and Burrill C. (1978). The training of co-ordination. *Arch phys. Med*; **59(12)**:567.

12. Basmajian J. V., ed. (1978). *Muscles Alive: Their Funtions Revealed by Electromyography*, 4th edn. Baltimore: Williams and Wilkins.

13. Taub E. and Berman A. J. (1968). Movement learning in the absence of sensory feedback. In *The Neuropsychology of Spatially Oriented Behavior* (Freedman S. J., ed.) pp. 173–192. Illinois: Dorsey Press.

14. Bobath B. (1978). *Adult Hemiplegia: Evaluation and Treatment*, 2nd edn. London: Heinemann Medical.

15. Riddock G. and Buzzard E. F. (1921). Reflex movements and postural reactions in quadriplegia, with special references to those of the upper limb. *Brain*; **44**:397.

16. Brunnstrom S. (1970). *Movement Therapy in Hemiplegia*. New York: Harper and Row.

17. Walsh F. M. R. (1923). Certain tonic or postural reflexes in hemiplegia with special reference to the so-called 'associated movements'. *Brain*; **1(46)**:1–37.

18. Eyzaguirre C. and Fidone S. J. (1975). *Physiology of the Nervous System*. Chicago: Year Book.

19. Phillips C. G. (1978). In laying the ghost of 'muscle versus ligaments', a lecture to the Xth Congress of Neurological Science. In *Muscles Alive; Their Functions Revealed by Electromyography*, 4th edn (Basmajian J. V., ed.) p. 107. Baltimore: Williams and Wilkins.

20. Knott M. and Voss D. E. (1968). *Proprioceptive Neuromuscular Facilitation*, 2nd edn. New York: Harper and Row.

21. Basmajian J. V. (1977). Motor learning and control: a working hypothesis. *Arch. Phys. Med. Rehabil*; **58**:38–41.

22. Norton B. J. and Sahrmann S. A. (1978). Reflex and voluntary electromyographic activity in patients with hemiparesis. *Phys. Ther*; **58**:951–5.

23. Taub E. (1980). Somato-sensory deafferentation research with monkeys: implications for rehabilitation medicine. In *Behavioral Psychology in Rehabilitation Medicine: Clinical Applications* (Ince L. P., ed.) pp. 371–401. Baltimore: Williams and Wilkins.

24. Anderson T. P. and Kottke F. J. (1978). Stroke rehabilitation: a reconsideration of some common attitudes. *Arch. phys. Med*; **59**:175–81.

25. Johnstone M. (1976). *The Stroke Patient: Principles of Rehabilitation*. London: Churchill Livingstone.

# Appendix 3

## Feedback

Feedback gives information about the environment and our place within it. It gives us knowledge of performance and knowledge of results. It is derived from external sources via the eyes, ears and skin, and from internal sources via proprioceptors and labyrinths. The term feedback is, however, also used to describe the generation of information within the brain itself, without direct reference to the periphery. It is considered that this allows for monitoring of movement, by a comparison between the intended motor output and the appropriate motor programme.

Kelso and Stelmach[1] categorise three types of feedback which are important in the modulation of movement as: (a) response feedback, in which information is received as a direct result of muscle contraction; (b) external feedback, where information is received from the environment usually in relation to a goal and as an indirect result of muscle contraction; and (c) internal feedback, or information generated prior to the response from structures within the nervous system.

**The relative importance of the various receptors to movement** and to the learning of movement is the subject of some controversy. The exact roles in motor control of muscle spindle[2,3] and Golgi tendon organ[4-6] and of the joint receptors[7-9] are not yet understood and results from studies remain conflicting. This situation reflects the complex nature of movement control.

It is possible that the emphasis which has been placed in physiotherapy on the importance of tactile and proprioceptive inflow may be misplaced.[10-14] Bizzi and Polit[15] comment that the proprioceptors have an uncertain role in the execution of voluntary movements. Taub and Berman[13] point out that although proprioceptive feedback may accompany movement, this does not mean it is essential to that movement. Jones[11] suggests that methods of physiotherapy to improve motor control may be ineffective if based solely on the theory that proprioceptive feedback is essential to movement.

The theory that somatosensory feedback is essential to movement was based largely on the work of Mott and Sherrington,[16] who showed in experiments with monkeys that, following complete deafferentation of one limb, the limb was in effect paralysed. The theory which developed from this was that tactile and proprioceptive impulses are essential for movement, that there could be no effective movement without such feedback.

However, several researchers, in particular Taub and his colleagues, have shown in their experiments with monkeys that following unilateral deafferentation, similar to that used in the original work by Mott and Sherrington, the animals can be induced to use the limb by training techniques and techniques to increase motivation, although the de-afferented animals needed more time to learn new tasks than the intact animals.[17] Furthermore, when monkeys are bilaterally deafferented,[13,18] following an immediate postoperative period when the limbs are useless, the animals are capable of using the limbs effectively for a wide variety of functions, without training, although they often lack the fluency of control and of precise timing found in intact animals.

The data from deafferentation experiments provide support for the theories of **central control of movement**. Evarts[19] points out that when sensory feedback is eliminated by deafferentation, it is interesting to see the extent to which new movements can be learned on the basis of knowledge of results and internal feedback. These studies and others imply that although sensory feedback is probably necessary for the fine tuning of movement, many motor programmes are genetically endowed, and peripheral feedback from movement itself is not as necessary as has been thought.

It may be that the central nervous system has a considerable amount of autonomy and independence from the periphery in the acquisition and maintenance of motor skill. The theory of internal feedback loops suggests that, once a motor skill is learned, the brain monitors its own efferent outflow, checking it against the appropriate motor programme.

In the last two decades, there has been a proliferation of theories regarding the role of central nervous system neurons in motor control. Terms such as feed forward,[20-23] efference copy,[24] corollary discharge[25-27] and central efferent monitoring[19,28,29] have been used in an attempt to explain the mechanisms which underly motor organisation. Miles and Evarts[30] discuss certain aspects of these motor organisation theories in an attempt to organise the data.

Herman[31] has suggested that the central nervous system appears to process and integrate spatial and temporal information which is derived from: (a) an intrinsic, centrally controlled sensori-motor loop which elicits signals of intended movement (central efferent monitoring), which could be called 'sense of innervation'; and (b) an extrinsic, peripherally controlled loop which elicits signals of actual movement, which could be called 'sense of performance'. Herman sums up the situation in this way: '. . . performance can be effectively controlled by the intrinsic system although external feedback may be continually required to distinguish finer levels of motor outflow discharges and to systematise information regarding the relationship between the two systems'.

Although the processes which underlie movement are not yet understood, it appears, therefore, that the central nervous system may be capable of generating and monitoring its own motor output, although somatosensory feedback is necessary at certain stages of motor learning and for certain motor acts if they are to be performed with a fine degree of accuracy. The role of the proprioceptors in motor control is being questioned and future experimental evidence will probably reveal more of their complex relationship with the brain.

Many studies have pointed out the relationship of vision to the acquisition and control of movement.[15,32,33] Other studies[11,34] have indicated that techniques of augmenting proprioceptive input such as resistance have little effect on accuracy of movement if verbal or visual knowledge of results is eliminated. It is probable that physiotherapists have not placed sufficient emphasis on, or perhaps realised the significance of, verbal feedback (particularly in relation to knowledge of performance), visual feedback and vestibular feedback to the learning of motor control.

It is important to be aware of the controversies surrounding motor control, as prognostic significance has been attached to sensory deficiencies following stroke, patients with somatosensory dysfunction being considered to do poorly in rehabilitation. Unfortunately, this assumption will result in a negative attitude towards such a patient.

It is the authors' experience that proprioceptive and tactile deficiencies are not necessarily indicators of poor prognosis following stroke. Poor results in rehabilitation and persistence of sensory dysfunction may be due instead to a failure of therapists to implement appropriate motor training techniques. The patient will learn effective movement again if knowledge of performance and of results,[35-37] via vision, hearing (verbal feedback) and manual guidance, are accurately and continually given to him by the therapist and if motivation is stimulated. Experience with the MRP indicates that proprioceptive, tactile and vestibular deficiencies gradually improve as therapy progresses, movement training itself apparently improving the patient's sensory perception. Movement is considered to be a vital factor in the brain's ability to adapt to visual, auditory, tactile and proprioceptive disturbance[38-40] and the MRP gives the patient early and active experience of familiar everyday movement with emphasis on the affected limbs. Treatment techniques which emphasise the intact limbs and do not give early practice of weight-bearing and early training of motor control in affected limbs probably augment and perpetuate disordered perception of sensation.

The following points about feedback should be kept in mind throughout the various sections of the MRP.

1. The patient is encouraged to use **visual feedback** to give him knowledge of performance and knowledge of results, and to provide him with spatial cues and to encourage scanning. He may need to be reminded to watch what he is doing, particularly with activities involving the hands. He is given the opportunity to compare his performance as he 'senses' it internally with what he looks like when he sees a videotape of himself, or when he compares his performance of the function with the therapist's demonstration. A patient with homonymous hemianopia may need to be reminded to turn his head to compensate for his deficit. However, specific visual defects related to stroke should be given special training.

2. The therapist gives **verbal feedback, as part of training,** continually monitoring the patient's performance so he knows whether or not it is correct, at what point the movement goes wrong, at what point inappropriate muscle activity is interfering with the movement. With very specific and accurate verbal feedback, patients following stroke can learn to recognise, isolate and produce fine degrees of neuromuscular activity.[31]

One segment of the MRP can be used as an example. In walking, one movement component to be learned is flexion of the knee at the start of swing phase, that is, with the hip in extension. This is practised in prone lying (see p. 133). Initially, the patient may only be able to contract his flexors spasmodically and in their inner range. The therapist feeds back to him information about muscle contraction immediately it occurs, getting him to practise eccentric and concentric movement in the small range he *can* control, gradually increasing this range. Verbal feedback must be instantaneous. As soon as the patient starts to lose control over the flexors, he should move back to the point where he has control, then gradually attempt to maintain that control over an increasing range of movement. The therapist must ensure that the patient can make the transition from concentric activity as he flexes his knee to eccentric activity as his leg is lowered into extension, and all of this activity must be monitored verbally to the patient as he moves.

This example illustrates what is probably a most important factor in the learning of movement. As Herman[31] has pointed out, motor control may be induced by providing a precise and reliable signal regarding the required function and the signal must provide information about the action with respect to the initiation, the execution and the termination of the action—and this without delay. The patient seems more readily able to learn the function if this information (by verbal feedback and manual guidance) is continued throughout his attempts at eliciting a controlled movement. As he develops control, feedback and guidance are gradually withdrawn.

**Verbal feedback is used carefully for reinforcement.** Only a successful performance, not merely a good attempt, is rewarded by 'Good', so the patient knows exactly what he must repeat. An unsuccessful performance should elicit from the therapist 'No, that's not right yet—try again, only this time make sure you don't move your other leg'.

Another important verbal technique in the MRP is the explanation to the patient of his problem, of what he is to practise and why. For him to relearn a component of movement such as flexion of the knee at the start of swing phase, he must have as complete an understanding as possible of the importance of this component in walking, and of the muscles he must activate in order to perform the component. By understanding the problem he is working on, the patient is able to make the best use of the verbal feedback he receives from the therapist as he practises controlling knee flexion and as he tries out his newly acquired control in the swing phase of walking.

Patients are frequently able to improve motor control with an explanation and verbal feedback as the only 'technique' used by the therapist. Unfortunately, some patients with communication problems will have difficulty with verbal techniques and these techniques must be replaced by non-verbal instruction and demonstrations, and by feedback given by gestures, photographs, or videotapes. Similarly, a patient with left brain damage may do better if verbal instructions are given **before** he attempts the task, not while he is performing it, as one process may interfere with the other.[41]

Other authors have expressed the view that the brain-damaged person would relearn more effective motor control if he received continuous accurate feedback as described above, and some have pointed out that physical therapy is usually deficient in this regard.[31] They have suggested, therefore, what is variously described as augmented feedback, sensory feedback, biological feedback therapy or biofeedback,[42-44] as a means of achieving this objective. Although, at the present time, biofeedback is mostly used where other methods of treatment have failed, or in conjunction with inappropriate and even conflicting methods of physiotherapy, it would provide a useful adjunct to the MRP because the Programme provides a specific analysis of motor problems and a guide to the muscles which need to be retrained. The limb load monitor has been used in conjunction with the standing sections in the Programme. Although biofeedback will no doubt be more effectively used in future rehabilitation, the value of feedback given by a skilled therapist, who understands normal movement and muscle action and who can analyse the patient's movement problems accurately and feed the appropriate information back to him, cannot be overemphasised. Biofeedback should be developed as a tool to enable the patient to undergo periods of monitored practice when the therapist is unavailable and for practice, with the therapist, of certain movement components or aspects of motor control with which he is having particular difficulty.

## REFERENCES

1. Kelso J. A. S. and Stelmach G. E. (1976). Central and peripheral mechanisms in motor control. In *Motor Control: Issues and Trends* (Stelmach G. E., ed.) New York: Academic Press.
2. Bizzi E., Polit A. and Morasso P. (1976). Mechanisms underlying achievement of final head position. *J. Neurophysiol*; **39**:435–44.
3. Kelso J. A. (1977). Motor control mechanisms underlying human movement reproduction. *J. Experimental Psychology: Human Perception and Performance*; 3:529–43(b).
4. Gelfan S. and Carter S. (1967). Muscle sense in man. *Exp. Neurol*; **18**:469–73.
5. Goodwin G. M., McCloskey D. I. and Matthews P. B. C. (1972). The contribution of muscle afferents to kinaesthesia shown by vibration-induced illusions of movement and by the effects of paralysing joint afferents. *Brain*; 95:705–748.
6. Matthews P. B. C. (1980). Developing views on the muscle spindle. In *Progress in Clinical Neurophysiology*, Vol. 8 (Desmedt J. E., ed.) pp. 12–27. Basel: Karger.

7. Skoglund S. (1973). Joint receptors and kinaesthesis. In *Handbook of Sensory Physiology: Somatosensory System 1* (Iggo I., ed.) pp. 111–136. Berlin: Springer.

8. Marteniuk R. G. (1979). Motor skill performance and learning: considerations for rehabilitation. *Physiotherapy Canada*; 31:4.

9. Roy E. A. and Williams I. D. (1979). Memory for location and extent: the influence of reduction of joint feedback information. In *Psychology of Motor Behaviour and Sport* (Roberts G. C., Newell K. M., eds.) Illinois: Human Kinetics Publishers.

10. Jones B. (1972). Outflow and inflow in movement duplication. *Perception and Psychophysics*; 12:95.

11. Jones B. (1974). The importance of memory traces of motor efferent discharge for learning skilled movements. *Develop. Med. Child Neurology*; 16:620–28.

12. Lashley K. S. (1964). *Brain Mechanisms and Intelligence*. New York: Hafner.

13. Taub E. and Berman A. J. (1968). Movement learning in the absence of sensory feedback. In *The Neuropsychology of Spatially Oriented Behavior* (Freedman S. J., ed.) pp. 173–192. Illinois: Dorsey Press.

14. Stelmach G. E. (1968). The accuracy of reproducing target positions under various tensions. *Psychonomic Science*; 13:287.

15. Bizzi E. and Polit A. (1979). Characteristics of the motor programs underlying visually evoked movements. In *Posture and Movement* (Talbott R. E. and Humphrey D. R., eds.) pp. 169–176. New York: Raven Press.

16. Mott F. W. and Sherrington C. S. (1895). Experiments upon the influence of sensory nerves upon movements and nutrition of the limbs. *Proc. roy. Soc. London*; 57:481–8.

17. Taub E. (1976). Motor behavior following deafferentation in the developing and motorically mature monkeys. In *Neural Control of Locomotion* (Herman R. *et al.*, eds.) pp. 675–705. New York: Plenum Press.

18. Taub E. (1980). Somatosensory deafferentation research with monkeys: implications for rehabilitation medicine. In *Behavioral Psychology in Rehabilitation Medicine: Clinical Implications* (Ince L. P., ed.) pp. 371–401. Baltimore: Williams and Wilkins.

19. Evarts E. V. (1971). Feedback and corollary discharge: a merging of the concepts. *Neurosciences Research Project Bulletin*; 9:86–112.

20. MacKay D. M. (1966). Cerebral organisation and the conscious control of action. In *Brain and Conscious Learning* (Eccles J. C., ed.) pp. 422–445. New York: Springer.

21. Ito M. (1974). The control mechanisms of cerebellar motor systems. In *The Neurosciences Third Study Program* (Schmitt F. O. and Worden F. G., eds.) pp. 293–303. Cambridge, Mass: MIT Press.

22. Kornhuber H. H. (1974). Cerebral cortex, cerebellum and basal ganglia: An introduction to their motor function. In *The Neurosciences Third Study Program* (Schmitt F. O. and Worden F. G., eds.) pp. 267–80. Cambridge, Mass: MIT Press.

23. Teuber H. L. (1974). Key problems in the programming of movements. *Brain Res*; 71:533–68.

24. Von Holst E. (1954). Relations between the central nervous system and peripheral organs. *Brit. J. anim. Behav*; 2:89.

25. Sperry R. W. (1950). Neural basis of the spontaneous optokinetic response produced by visual inversion. *J. Comp. physiol. Psychol*; 43:482–9.

26. Teuber H. L. (1964). The riddle of frontal lobe function in man. In *The Frontal Granular Cortex and Behavior* (Warren J. M. and Akert K., eds.) pp. 410–444. New York: McGraw Hill.

27. Kennedy D. and Davis W. J. (1977). Organisation of invertebrate motor

systems. *Handb. Physiol*; 1:1023–87.

28. Oscarsson O. (1970). Functional organisation of spino-cerebellar paths. In *Handbook of Sensory Physiology 2* (Iggo A., ed.) pp. 121–127. Berlin: Springer.

29. Bruner J. S. (1973). Organisation of early skilled action. *Child Development*; **44**,4:1 11.

30. Miles F. A. and Evarts E. V. (1979). Concepts of motor organisation. *Ann. Rev. Psychol*; **30**:327 62.

31. Herman R. (1973). Augmented sensory feedback in the control of limb movement. In *Neural Organisation and its Relevance to Prosthetics, Symposia Specialists*; **73–82041**:197–212.

32. Smyth M. M. (1978). Attention to visual feedback and motor learning. *Journal of Motor Behaviour*; **10**:185–90.

33. Adams J. A., Gopher D. and Lintern G. (1977). Effects of visual and proprioceptive feedback on motor learning. *J. exp. Psychol*; **9**:11–22.

34. William I. D. and Stelmach G. E. (1968). The accuracy of reproducing target positions under various tensions. *Psychonomic Science*; **13**:287.

35. Gentile A. M. (1972). A working model of skill acquisition with application to teaching. *Quest*; **17**:3–23.

36. Marteniuk R. G. (1976). *Information Processing in Motor Skills*. New York: Holt, Rinehart and Winston.

37. Wallace S. A. and Hagler R. W. (1979). Knowledge of performance and the learning of a closed motor skill. *Res. Quart*; **50**,2:265–71.

38. Held R. (1965). Plasticity in sensory motor systems. *Scientific American*; **213**:84–94.

39. Luria A. R. (1961). *The Role of Speech in the Regulation of Normal and Abnormal Behaviour*. Oxford: Pergamon.

40. Greenwald A. G. (1970). Sensory feedback mechanism in performance control: with special reference to ideo-motor mechanism. *Psychol. Rev*; **77**:73–99.

41. Stockmeyer S. (1981). Interference and Co-operation in Hemispheric Function. Unpublished paper given at *First Austral-Asian Physiotherapy Congress, Singapore*.

42. Brudny J., Korein J., Grynbaum B. and Sachs-Frankel G. (1977). Sensory feedback therapy in patients with brain insult. *Scand. J. Rehab. Med*; **9**:155–63.

43. Gonella C., Kalish R. and Hale G. (1978). A commentary on electromyographic feedback in physical therapy. *Phys. Ther*; **58**:11–14.

44. Kelly J. L., Baker M. P. and Wolf S. L. (1979). Procedures for E. M. G. biofeedback training in involved upper extremities of hemiplegic patients. *Phys. Ther*; **59**,12:1500–1507.

# *Appendix 4*

# *Practice*

Practice is known to be a necessary prerequisite for acquiring skill in movement. Practice without any other consideration, however, is not necessarily effective nor will it necessarily result in learning. For example, without feedback as to its accuracy or otherwise, practice may actually prevent the learning of skill. Some factors which must be considered if practice is to be effective in rehabilitation are outlined below.

## GOAL IDENTIFICATION

Learning a complex motor skill involves two major components: identifying what is to be learned and organising the information in the correct sequence to carry out the task. The patient must be aware of the goal for which he is practising and the goal must be readily identifiable as one which he considers important. The goal should be short term, that is, capable of fulfilment on the day of practice, although it will be directly related to another, longer term, goal. For example, the short-term goal may be to straighten the hip in standing; the longer term goal would be to stand alone or to walk.

A goal should, at all stages of the patient's rehabilitation, be reasonably hard yet attainable. This usually produces a better performance than a goal which is too easy or too general.[1] When the patient is practising with the therapist, he should experience success, even if at first his performance needs substantial manual guidance and monitoring from the therapist. He should not repeatedly experience failure. He should finish each therapy session with the feeling that he has been practising successfully and that he will continue to be successful with less and less guidance. As soon as he performs correctly, and sometimes it is more effective just before this point, the therapist adds increasing complexity to what he is performing or slightly varies the task. For example, the patient's goal may be to stand erect and make the necessary postural adjustments. Once he can achieve this, even though not 100% of the time or with 100% accuracy, the therapist suggests a new goal. The patient now has to turn his body and look behind him without moving his feet. Although he has a different goal, in fact he is still practising making postural adjustments, but the therapist has added variety and complexity to the task.

Variety and complexity can also be added by changing the rhythm or the timing of a movement. Practising in this way should enable the patient to push his optimum performance continually higher. A major fault in much therapy is that the patient spends time practising what he can already do. As Taub[2] suggests, it is important that when the patient is ready he moves on, as practising at the same level of performance may actually impede progress.

Similarly, the goal can be changed, the timing or rhythm altered, in order to make a task possible if the patient is having difficulty practising without error. To go back to the above example, if the patient is having difficulty making postural adjustments, and is making too many errors, the therapist may change the goal, asking the patient to put his hands on her shoulders and to shift his pelvis laterally 2·5 cm (1 in) to one side and then to the other, or forward (see Fig. 8.14a). His goal is now to exercise conscious control of his trunk on his legs in preparation for standing alone and making postural adjustments automatically. Note that it is only the short-term goal which has changed. Analysis of the reasons he is having difficulty has enabled the therapist to determine the action to be taken. It would have been incorrect of her to assume that standing is too difficult for the patient and to postpone the goal of standing balance in favour of some activity in sitting.

## RELEVANCE OF PRACTICE

The patient must be able to see the immediate relevance of what he is practising to the functions he wants to perform. However, in much present-day rehabilitation, the patient practises what is not directly relevant, for example leg and trunk exercises on his back, exercises on the floor, exercises for his intact side and gross movement patterns for his limbs and trunk.[3–5] Such exercises do not convey to the learner the dynamic components which are necessary if he is to perform those everyday functions which he must learn.[6] Rehabilitation should be more directly related to everyday life. The MRP consists of modules of everyday activities in order to prepare the patient for what he needs to do in his daily life and for what will be expected of him. Practice sessions simulate real-life situations and make the adjustment from the therapeutic session to everyday life relatively easy.

The stimulation of recovering muscle activity must be relevant to function.[7] Neither the therapist nor the patient should be aiming at eliciting indiscriminate muscle activity. Exercises to improve muscle activity are frequently given without any consideration of how the muscle would work in a particular function. This is a waste of the patient's time and will result in him learning incorrect movement habits. If he has difficulty contracting his knee extensors when weight-bearing through the leg (i.e. in 0–15° in standing or during the stance phase of walking), he will not learn to control them for this activity by practising full-range knee extension. He may learn to contract his knee extensors in their outer range but still be unable to control the necessary 0–15° of knee movement when bearing weight in standing (i.e. with the foot as a fixed point). Instead, the patient needs to practise concentric and eccentric knee extension activity in the 0–15° range with pressure through the leg to mimic the effect of the body weight in standing (see p. 127).

Similarly, it may be possible to elicit foot dorsiflexion in sitting (i.e. with hip and knee flexed) but the patient may find it impossible to dorsiflex his foot on heel strike (i.e. with hip flexed and knee extended). The patient should practise this muscle activity in a manner which is relevant to what is required for the particular function (see Fig. 8.19). Practice must therefore take into account the influence of gravity, leverage and joint position.

Practice should seem logical to the patient, the various steps following each other in a systematic order. He needs to understand what he is doing. Throughout each part of the MRP, the patient should see the logical sequence of what he is practising now in terms of what he will do next. If the material is well organised, he will be able to store it in an organised manner for retrieval when necessary. The therapist should remember that familiar tasks are probably learned and retained better than unusual ones. Similarly, there is a greater transference of training when preparatory activities contain components identical to those required for the performance of the skill itself.[6]

## WHOLE OR PART PRACTICE

It is generally considered that motor acts can be taught in their entirety or broken down into their component parts.[1] Which is the better method has been discussed in the literature on motor learning in relation to non brain-damaged people.[8,9] Although it may be sufficient for the stroke patient to practise an entire activity, such as standing up from a chair, it is usually necessary for him to undergo some preparation. The activity is broken down into its component parts and the patient practises those with which he is having difficulty. He may need to practise contracting specific muscles or muscle groups. He should practise each component in the sequence in which it normally occurs and practice of the component is followed immediately by practice of the entire activity. Using the example above, the patient practises inclining his extended trunk forward at his hips in order to get his centre of gravity appropriately placed for standing up. This constitutes practice of a component. He must then practise standing up from the chair, concentrating on the component and thinking about where it goes in the sequence of activity. He should have the opportunity to repeat the practice of any component he finds difficult whenever necessary and whenever unwanted movement habits are retarding progress.

## ATTENTIVENESS

Initially, the patient may have difficulty isolating the muscle action required, or a particular component in an activity. He will need to be reminded to concentrate and be attentive to what he is doing. If too much information is given to him, he may pay attention to what is irrelevant. Clinically, inattentiveness or misdirected attention is found to limit the effectiveness of practice and Diller[10] reports that improved performance has been found to be associated with improved attention.

The therapist should make an active attempt to engage in eye contact while within relatively close range of the patient, as this not only aids concentration but also orientation in space. Furthermore, it is a means of communicating positive attitudes[11] and helps create a bond between therapist and patient. Early practice of balance in sitting with emphasis on eye and head control seems to foster the ability to pay attention and to concentrate. This is probably due to the regaining of movement control in a position which enables the patient to re-orient himself with his surroundings. The sitting position also enables eye contact and therefore communication with staff and relatives.

## CUES

Different cues are probably more important at different stages of learning.[1,12] Fitts[13] suggested three stages in learning a skill—cognitive, associative and automatic. The patient seems often to respond best in early recovery to more cognitive cues. However, once he has developed some motor control he may respond better to more automatic ones. One of the objectives of practice is to enable him to make the transition from the cognitive stage to the automatic stage.

Verbal and visual cues appear to be essential in the early stages of learning. What the therapist says to the patient before and during practice constitutes an important **verbal cue**, and instructions and explanations need to be very direct and explicit in order to trigger off the desired response. For example, 'Move your bottom back and sit down' may be more effective in initiating hip and knee flexion with weight shift backwards than 'Sit down' or 'Bend your knees and hips'.

Sometimes, in order to elicit the desired response, the therapist may need to give the patient a different goal (by verbal cue or instruction), although *her* goal remains the same. For example, if the therapist is teaching the patient to extend his hip in lying in preparation for standing with his hips in normal alignment, she may ask him to contract his hip extensors (see Fig. 7.8b). If he cannot do this, she gives him another goal (i.e. changes the verbal cue), which would have the same result, asking him to push his heel down towards the floor, thus directing his attention away from the specific muscle activity. When he is successful, she takes him back to his former goal, pointing out that he has in fact achieved what she had originally asked.

The therapist must take care not to give so lengthy an instruction that the patient does not know at what part of the sentence to direct his attention. She should ensure, for example, that the essential verbal cue does not come at the end of a long sentence, by which time a patient who is having difficulty concentrating will have stopped listening. Similarly, she should not distract a patient who is having difficulty shifting from one topic to another by introducing irrelevant information. She should also take care to avoid information overload.

**Visual cues** are important, particularly in the early stages of learning, for directing and correcting movement. The eyes give information on position in space and position relative to other objects. For example, the patient reaches towards the therapist's hand, or turns to look behind him. The therapist must be prepared to guide and encourage eye movement just as she would guide and encourage other movements. Many stroke patients, particularly those with right brain damage, have great difficulty initially in directing their gaze to the appropriate place and keeping it there.

Used discretely, **tactile cues** will reinforce verbal instruction. However, persistent tactile stimulation will distract the patient's attention from the activity he is practising. It is important to reduce all tactile stimuli to the most essential[10] so the patient can concentrate only on the cues which are relevant. That is, the most essential cues should not be lost amidst a variety of different ones. If the patient has tactile inattention (extinction), it is particularly important that tactile stimulation to the intact side is minimal until he has been trained to overcome his tendency to extinguish the stimulus on the affected side.

## PRACTICE WITHOUT ERROR

Practice of an incorrect movement will retard progress, as the patient will, at a later stage, have to unlearn the incorrect movements in order to learn the activity correctly. Errors, if they are practised and become well-learned responses, interfere with subsequent attempts at making a correct response. It is known that if an athlete practises a motor skill incorrectly, he will have to spend considerable time unlearning the abnormal movement in order to be able to perform it correctly.[14] The stroke patient will have even greater difficulty because of his tendency to develop the wrong emphasis in movement and also because it will usually be too frustrating and complex for him to learn to move in a different manner once he has learned incorrectly. Consequently, if, for example, the patient practises walking with a three- or four-point cane or with a wide base, he will be practising abnormal walking and it is unlikely that he will be able to unlearn this pattern later and learn to walk correctly. Also, if he has a low expectation of his motor potential he may no longer *want* to make the change. Lack of success in rehabilitation may well stem from a failure to understand the ineffectiveness and the falsity of the independence which results from a compensation with the intact side at the expense of recovery of the affected side.

Unfortunately, compensation with the intact side may reinforce another problem, what Taub[2] calls 'learned non-use'. In the example given above, the patient who learns to walk with a four-point cane will not take weight normally through his affected leg and, because he does not *need* to use this leg correctly in walking, he will learn *not* to. Clinically it is very apparent that, although a person may, if he is motivated to do so, be able to unlearn an incorrect movement and learn to perform it correctly, it is usually impossible to overcome 'learned non-use' of a limb, probably due to secondary perceptual dysfunction.

## PATIENT PARTICIPATION

The patient must be encouraged and shown how to develop a problem-solving attitude to practice by questioning his performance, comparing it to normal and correcting errors when they occur. He should work with the therapist in evaluating his performance and learn from her his major problems and the strategies which he can use to overcome them. He needs to know why he fails and why he succeeds and what solutions are available for overcoming error. He should **actively** participate and not just have things done to him and for him.

**Mental practice** or **task rehearsal**[15–17] appears to be helpful to some patients in learning particular movements and can be used even before the person has regained the ability to elicit active muscle contraction. For specific periods of time during the day, the patient thinks through a movement, visualising the entire movement in his mind. As with physical practice, mental practice should be performed without error. As this is difficult to monitor, the therapist should ensure that the patient knows accurately the movements he will practise. They should be few in number and simple in execution.

## AUGMENTED PRACTICE

Although the most meaningful and effective practice sessions for the stroke patient in terms of learning will be those he spends with his therapist, it is important to consider what happens for the rest of the day, as actual physical therapy sessions will occupy only a small part of the 24 hours. The need for consistency throughout the day, with the patient having the opportunity to practise particular skills with other members of the staff, has been discussed elsewhere in this book (see p. 12). However, some skills will not be practised between therapy sessions and therefore the repetition of accurate, near-peak performance, which is necessary for the development of movement control, does not take place.[18] Physical practice may be augmented, both with and without the therapist's presence, by videotapes[19] illustrating normal performance of the skill he is learning, the opportunity to see his own performance, photographs of incorrect and correct performance and biofeedback (see p. 158).

Programmed instruction by videotape is a useful adjunct to treatment, enabling the patient to use visual instruction as an additional guide to learning and to enable him to check up on his mental practice. A study by Gonnella *et al.*[6] demonstrated that self-instruction using an audiovisual medium was effective in enabling normal subjects to learn a new skill. The hypothesis that subjects could learn the cognitive aspects of the motor skill in one viewing of a film was supported, and transfer of learning to the physical performance of the skill was found to occur.

## FATIGUE

The therapist need not assume that the patient, because he has had a stroke or because he is elderly, will tire easily during practice. If he appears to be fatigued , or complains of fatigue, the possible reasons for this must be considered. It may be that he is having too much sedation or that his vital capacity is reduced. The activities he is expected to practise may be too difficult, in which case he may appear 'unco-operative', or too easy, in which case he becomes bored and dispirited. He may not be able to see the immediate relevance of what he is practising. It is interesting that the patient who is experiencing success during therapy sessions and whose programme enables him to move on from one task to the next, seldom complains of fatigue. The normal fatigue which accompanies physical activity will respond to a period of rest, and fatigue within normal limits does not affect learning, although it may temporarily affect performance.[20-22].

After the patient has been practising a particular task for a period of time, the resultant fatigue is probably related to one or other of the following factors: (a) mental—the necessity to concentrate hard on a particular action; and (b) physical—the muscle activity necessary to maintain a position and to move. It is more effective in terms of the patient's need to learn if he is given another activity to practise rather than given a 'rest'. A different activity will require different muscle work and a different goal on which to concentrate. It seems necessary to keep up the person's level of alertness and to transfer the alertness developed in one activity to another activity. It was found in studies with normal subjects[23,24] that the amount of muscle work which could be performed after a 'diverting activity' was always greater than the amount of muscle work which could be performed after a passive pause. One study with a small group of patients[25] indicates that this may also be so following stroke.

## REFERENCES

1. Singer R. N. (1980). *Motor Learning and Human Performance*, 3rd edn. New York: Macmillan.
2. Taub E. (1980). Somatosensory deafferentation research with monkeys: implications for rehabilitation medicine. In *Behavioral Psychology in Rehabilitation Medicine: Clinical Application* (Ince L. P., ed.) pp. 371–401. Baltimore: Williams and Wilkins.

3. Brunnstrom S. (1970). *Movement Therapy in Hemiplegia*. New York: Harper and Row.
4. Knott M. and Voss D. E. (1968). *Proprioceptive Neuromuscular Facilitation*, 2nd edn. New York: Harper and Row.
5. Johnstone M. (1978). *Restoration of Motor Function in the Stroke Patient*. London: Churchill Livingstone.
6. Gonnella C., Hale G., Ionta M. and Perry J. C. (1981). Self-instruction in a perceptual motor skill. *Phys. Ther*; **61**:177–84.
7. Basmajian J. V. (1977). Motor learning and control: a working hypothesis. *Arch. phys. Med*; **58**:38–41.
8. Naylor J. C. and Briggs C. E. (1963). Long-term retention of learned skills: A review of the literature. *ASD Technical Report* **61–390**. US Department of Commerce.
9. Fitts P. M. and Posner M. I. (1967). *Human Performance*. Belmont, California: Brooks/Cole.
10. Diller L. (1970). Psychomotor and vocational rehabilitation. In *Behavioral Change in Cerebrovascular Disease* (Benton A. L., ed.) pp. 81–116. New York: Harper and Row.
11. Mehrabian A. (1969). Significance of posture and position in the communication of attitude and status relationships. *Psychol. Bull*; **71**:359–72.
12. Leithwood K. A. and Fowler W. (1971). Complex motor learning in four-year olds. *Child Develop*; **42**:781–92.
13. Fitts P. M. (1964). Perceptual motor skill learning. In *Categories of Human Learning* (Melton A. W., ed.) pp. 243–286. New York: Academic Press.
14. Lawther J. D. (1977). *The Learning and Performance of Physical Skills*, 2nd edn. Englewood Cliffs, New Jersey: Prentice Hall.
15. Jacobsen E. (1932). Muscular phenomenon during imagining. *Amer. J. Psychol*; **49**:677–94.
16. Jones G. J. (1965). Motor learning without demonstration of physical practice, under two conditions of mental practice. *Res. Quart*; **36**:270–76.
17. Cardinall N. (1977). Mental practice. Unpublished paper delivered at *53rd Congress of APTA, St Louis, Missouri*.
18. Leiper C., Miller A., Lang J. and Herman R. (1981). Sensory feedback for head control in cerebral palsy. *Phys. Ther*; **61**:512–18.
19. Del Rey P. (1971). The effects of video-taped feedback on form accuracy and latency in an open and closed environment. *J. Motor Behavior*; **3**:281–7.
20. Marteniuk R. G. (1979). Motor skill performance and learning: considerations for rehabilitation. *Physiotherapy Canada*; **31**:187–202.
21. Bilodeau E. A. (1952). Massing and spacing phenomena as functions of prolonged and extended practice. *J. exp. Psychol*; **44**:108–13.
22. Cochran B. J. (1975). Effect of physical fatigue on learning to perform a novel motor task. *Res. Quart*; **46**:243–249.
23. Asmussen E. and Mazin B. (1978). A central nervous component in local muscular fatigue. *Europ. J. appl. Physiol*; **38**:9–15.
24. Asmussen E. and Mazin B. (1978). Recuperation after muscle fatigue by 'diverting activities'. *Europ. J. appl. Physiol*; **38**:1–7.
25. Chaco J., Blank A. and Gonen B. (1981). Recovery after muscular fatigue in hemiparesis. *Amer. J. phys. Med*; **60**:30–32.

# Appendix 5

# Adjustments to gravity

Balance is essential in the maintenance of all positions and the execution of all movements. The physiological mechanisms thought to control balance are described in the literature.[1-3]

The human body is perpetually submitted to the force of gravity. The whole motor system is organised towards counteracting the effects of this force, both when the body is immobile and when it is moving. We can only discount the force of gravity when we are lying down or sitting with the body fully supported. Holt[4] comments that, because it cannot be seen, we sometimes forget the effect of gravity on everything we do. This is probably one of the reasons why detection of balance problems in patients is relatively difficult and balance problems are frequently analysed incorrectly.

The **force of gravity** is always exerted in a vertical direction downwards towards the centre of the earth. The line which passes from the centre of gravity of the mass towards the centre of the earth is known as the **line of gravity**. A mass is said to be balanced when its **centre of gravity** is positioned over the base of support and the centre of gravity is the point about which the mass balances, that is, the point at which the weight of the mass can be considered to be controlled. In general, it is said that the centre of gravity of the body is in the region of the hips.[5] (Under static conditions it is estimated that the centre of gravity lies just anterior to the second sacral vertebra.[6]) The human body consists of segments which are constantly moving and different in shape from each other. The 'shape' of the human body is constantly changing during movement, and its centre of gravity will therefore also change.

The **ability to maintain an upright position** (i.e. a posture) involves some postural movements to protect the stability of the body. These movements are **automatic** and in general they occur below the level of consciousness. In other words, the subject is unaware of them. Usually they are adjustments of the body segments on one another and do not move the body from one position to another. These adjustments generally involve muscular activity throughout the body even though the adjustments may be slight, and Martin[7] comments that they are in keeping with the principles of mechanics.

Most volitional movements contain a substrate of automatic postural adjustment. When a subject is moving from one position to another, for example transferring from sitting to standing, he may be conscious of the activity and the purpose of the activity, yet throughout the act there are supporting and balancing activities of which he remains unaware. Volitional movement of the hands requires not only postural fixation of the shoulder but also subtle postural movements which occur below the level of consciousness in order to adjust to the alteration in the centre of gravity which results from the arm movement. Some authors suggest that this adjustment is anticipatory in that the centre of gravity is shifted before the movement takes place. Massion and Gahery[8] cite several references to support this.

The maintenance of standing posture is associated with **postural sway**, which involves little muscular activity. When the subject is standing at ease, postural sway is only slight. Herman[9] states that 'the ability of man to stand with little expenditure of neuromuscular energy is due to the tensile strength of ligaments and muscles, the mechanical features of some joints and the compensatory changes of the centre of gravity of body segments'. He goes on, 'the control of balance in posture is to provide intermittent correction of balance rather than steady antigravitational control'. Balance in standing must be maintained in both an antero-posterior plane and a lateral plane. To allow for normal body sway in standing without loss of balance, weight should fall near the centre of the base, between the feet and in front of the ankles. The normal base in standing is with the feet a few inches apart as they are when the legs are vertical. This gives as large a base as possible without introducing a diagonal force against the ground.

In simple terms, **postural movements keep the body segments appropriately aligned**. Efficient balance requires correct timing and muscular control in order to maintain alignment. If a body segment is out of line with the segment(s) below, the bones and the joints are out of line, tension of the opposing ligaments is unbalanced and excessive muscle tension is required to prevent loss of balance. Normally, body balance is maintained with a minimum of strain when each segment is centred over the one below, i.e. normally aligned. **Body segments are constantly moving**. Whenever a segment moves, there is an unconscious adjustment of the body. Postural changes have been observed even during movements of the thoracic walls during respiration. When a body part moves away from the line of gravity in one direction, there is a shift in the centre of gravity in the same direction. Another segment must therefore move in the opposite direction. If the arms are lifted forward to shoulder level, the centre of gravity is now further forward and upward within the body, and the adjustment of the body is backwards. Just how great the adjustment is depends on the weight of the arms and the distance they are moved. If the subject has a weight in his hand, the adjustment of the body will be greater. If the displacement is great, there must be considerable adjustment in the opposite direction to keep the centre of gravity over the base. This involves not only movement of the trunk and head but also movement of the limbs in order to preserve balance.

If the line of gravity falls outside the base and appropriate adjustment can no longer be made, a new base directly below the centre of gravity must be established. In other words, balance is lost at this point until a new base is established. **Loss of balance**, therefore, occurs when the person is unable to compensate and to preserve balance. At this point the limbs are extended to absorb the impact (protective support).

**Balance training** should not be considered as separate from training in everyday activities. Balance is dynamic, it is never static, and balance training should enable the learner to regain the dynamic components necessary for each individual function. Balance may, in certain circumstances, be improved without direct training, being acquired dynamically as part of the practice of a function.[10]

The principles of stimulation of balance in the MRP are based on an understanding of the fundamental effects of gravity and the body's anticipated responses to these effects. These principles are as follows.

1. The maintenance of stability in the upright position requires very little neuromuscular energy when body segments are aligned correctly. Emphasis in treatment is therefore on correcting alignment of body segments with a normal base of support and stimulating the slight adjustments which make up postural sway. Resisted isometric contractions are contra-indicated in treatment because they elicit an abnormal amount of muscle activity and interfere with the training of the subtle adjustments involved in normal posture sway.

2. Movement or displacement of any segment of the body is a source of disequilibrium because of the shift of the centre of gravity which must be accompanied by an appropriate adjustment of posture, i.e. compensatory movements of body segments in an opposite direction to rebalance the body. The patient must be trained to make these adjustments himself as he moves from one position to another or as he moves one body segment. He will need to do this at a cognitive level at first, but the objective is to establish responses which are automatic.

3. The retraining of balance in sitting and standing requires that the patient experience these positions. That is, he will not regain the ability to balance in standing until he is in the standing position. It should be noted that the regaining of balance control in sitting is not a prerequisite for balancing in standing. The alignment of the body segments to each other in sitting and standing is different and therefore the muscle activity is also different. It is important to recognise the fact that the patient will only regain good control over balance in either position if he practises in that position. Lawther[11] cites several studies which indicate that balance is highly specific in terms of particular activities and positions.

4. During treatment, the therapist must ensure that she does not position herself too closely to the patient or hold him in such a way that she will inhibit the body's automatic adjustment to shifts in the centre of gravity.

# REFERENCES

1. Eyzaguirre C. and Fidone S. J. (1975). *Physiology of the Nervous System*, 2nd edn. Chicago: Year Book Medical Publishers.
2. Daube J. R. and Sandbok B. A. (1978). *Medical Neurosciences: An Approach to Anatomy, Pathology and Physiology by Systems and Levels*. Boston: Little Brown.
3. Guyton A. C. (1980). *Textbook of Medical Physiology*, 6th edn. Philadelphia: W. B. Saunders.
4. Holt K. S., ed. (1975). How and why children move. In *Movement and Child Development*, pp. 1–7. Philadelphia: W. B. Saunders.
5. Broer M. R. and Zernicke R. F. (1979). *Efficiency of Human Movement*, 4th edn. Philadelphia: W. B. Saunders.
6. Saunders J. B., Inman V. T. and Eberhart H. D. (1953). The major determinant in normal and pathological gait. *J. Bone Jt Surg*; **35-A**:543–58.
7. Purdon Martin J. (1977). A short essay on posture and movement, *J. Neurol. Neurosurg. Psychiat*; **40**:25–9.
8. Massion J. and Gahery Y. (1979). Diagonal stance in quadrupeds: a postural support for movement. In *Progress in Brain Research*, 50 (Granit R. and Pompeiano O., eds.) pp. 219–26. Amsterdam: Elsevier/North Holland Biomedical Press.
9. Herman R. (1976). Postural control and therapeutic implications. In *Advances in Orthotics* (Murdoch G., ed.) pp. 471–483. London: Edward Arnold.
10. Gonella C., Hale G., Ionta M. and Perry J. C. (1981). Self-instruction in a perceptual motor skill. *Phys. Ther*; **61**:177–84.
11. Lawther J. D. (1977). *The Learning and Performance of Physical Skills*, 2nd edn. Englewood Cliffs, New Jersey: Prentice Hall.

# Index